MEDICAL CIRCUMCISION AND HIV/AIDS POLICY

MEDICAL CIRCUMCISION AND HIV/AIDS POLICY

JAMES KITYO

Bethesda Scientific

London – Washington
Academica Press

Library of Congress Cataloging-in-Publication Data

Names: Kityo, James, author.
Title: Medical circumcision and HIV/AIDS policy / James Kityo.
Description: London ; Washington : Bethesda Scientific, Academica Press,
[2019] | Includes bibliographical references and index.
Identifiers: LCCN 2018059579 | ISBN 9781680534856 (hardcover : alk. paper)
Subjects: | MESH: HIV Infections--prevention & control | Acquired
Immunodeficiency Syndrome--prevention & control | Circumcision, Male |
Treatment Outcome | Health Policy | Uganda
Classification: LCC RA643.8 | NLM WC 503.6 | DDC 614.5/99392--dc23
LC record available at https://lccn.loc.gov/2018059579

DEDICATION

This piece of academic work is dedicated to my late uncle *Ensi-Egula-Mirambo* (RIP), of Kazo Bwaise, Kampala, who died this year 2007 at the age of 95. This work is a reminder of his great valour exhibited in World War II in Burma, India and Kenya.

And to my mother, Margaret Masolo and Daddy, Augustine Peter Labongo, for paying my school fees up to high school and bringing me up as a humble child.

Also dedicated to my wife Marie Namuyanja (Pine); our daughters Precious Namayanja and Juliet Nambwere.

Finally, to my sisters; Jeska, Ruth and Night for taking care of mummy during my time in the UK.

.

ACKNOWLEDGEMENTS

Firstly, I acknowledge the Ford Foundation International, for having identified me from a remote village of Mbirizi in Masaka and offered me a scholarship to pursue further studies in the UK.

Secondly, I thank the entire academic and support staff of the Nuffield Institute for Health. I acknowledge that my interaction with members of staff, has initiated me into the thinking process. I am particularly humbled by the skills and analytical approaches to public health issues, which I have gained.

Thirdly, I thank my supervisor, Kamran Saddiqi for giving me an opportunity to think and write.

Fourthly, I thank my adopted family in Leeds – Ricky's family. I felt so much at home. I pray that the Almighty blesses, Canvir, Khaya, Mintri and Ricky.

Fifthly, I thank teacher Reinhard Huss, for reinvigorating my interest in the environment, especially the need for us to think about our individual responsibilities on the environment.

I also thank Philippa Bird, for contacting and reassuring my family during her assignments in Uganda.

I thank John Cowe, my language teacher, at the Leeds Language Centre, for all the guidance during the language course, which helped me improve on my Ugandan English.

Special thanks also go to Herman Butime, Miriam Scherer, MaryRose Kahwa Giatas and Halimah Yunus, for their invaluable ideas about my topic.

I thank Group one (2006) Leeds language class - Imad, Andrej, Miriam, Anne, Yuko, Heejoan, Migumi, Makiko, Hee – Up, Aki and Germana for all the films, fun and parties, while in Leeds.

Finally, I thank the HMPP class for all the discussions and academic fraternity that enabled me to learn.

TABLE OF CONTENTS

GENERAL INTRODUCTION 1

INTRODUCTION 1
JUSTIFICATION OF THE STUDY 1
PROBLEM IDENTIFICATION 2
PROBLEM ANALYSIS 3
AIM OF THE STUDY 4
OBJECTIVES OF THE STUDY 5
METHODOLOGY 5
THE STUDY AREA 5
SOURCES OF DATA 5
STAKE HOLDERS 8
SCOPE 8
THE OUTPUT 9
THE ROLE OF THE AUTHOR 9
OUTLINE OF THE DISSERTATION 10
CONCLUSION 11

1. CHAPTER ONE 13

1.1. INTRODUCTION 13
1.2. GENERAL DEMOGRAPHIC DATA 13
1.3. HIV/AIDS IN UGANDA 14
1.4. DETERMINANTS AND CONSEQUENCES 15
1.4.1. CULTURAL PRACTICES AND ATTITUDES 15
1.4.2. LONG TERM IMPACT OF HIV/AIDS 17
1.4.3. ROLE OF RELIGIOUS BODIES IN HEALTH 17
1.4.4. POLITICAL ORGANISATION AND HIV/AIDS 18
1.4.5. THE HEALTH INFRASTRUCTURE 18
1.4.6. HUMAN RESOURCES FOR HEALTH 21
1.4.7. SOURCES OF FUNDING FOR HIV/AIDS 22
1.5. CURRENT HIV/AIDS INITIATIVES 22
1.6. RELIGIOUS BARRIERS TO HIV/AIDS PROGRAMME 23
1.7. POLITICAL BARRIERS 24
1.8. CORRUPTION 25

1.9. CONCLUSION 25

2. CHAPTER TWO 27

2.1 HIV/AIDS, SEXUAL HEALTH POLICIES AND MC 27
2.2 INTRODUCTION 27
2.3 DEFINITION OF POLICY 29
2.4 BACKGROUND TO UGANDA'S HIV/AIDS POLICY 29
2.5 THE BEHAVIOURAL APPROACH 32
2.5.1 ABSTINENCE 33
2.5.2 FAITHFULNESS 34
2.5.3 CONDOMS 34
2.6 STIs 37
2.7 VCT SERVICES 38
2.8 IEC 40
2.9 ART AND PMTCT 40
2.10 CONCLUSION 40

3. CHAPTER THREE 43

3.1 OPPORTUNITIES AND CHALLENGES OF MC 43
3.2 INTRODUCTION 43
3.3 WHAT IS MC? 43
3.4 OPPORTUNITIES PROVIDED BY MC 44
3.4.1 THE MEDICAL TRIALS ON MC 44
3.4.2 CHALLENGES NOTED FROM RCTs 47
3.4.3 POLICY IMPLICATIONS 47
3.4.4 EFFECTIVENESS OF MC FROM SYSTEMATIC REVIEWS 48
3.4.5 MC FROM A WIDER SOCIAL ECONOMIC CONTEXT 49
3.4.6 NEONATAL MC 51
3.4.7 ACCEPTABILITY OF MC IN COMMUNITIES 52
3.4.8 ACCEPTABILITY OF MC AMONG WOMEN 53
3.4.9 INTERNATIONAL ACCEPTANCE OF MC 54
3.5 CHALLENGES 57
3.5.1 THE COSTS OF PROVIDING MMC 57
3.5.2 CONSENT, ETHICAL PRACTICE AND HUMAN RIGHTS 58
3.6 CONCLUSION 60

4. CHAPTER FOUR 63

4.1. INTRODUCTION 63
4.2. MMC AND HIV/AIDS POLICY OPTIONS FOR CONSIDERATION 63
4.3. NEONATAL MC 64
4.4. MMC AND ABC (14 - 24 YEARS) 65
4.5. TARGETED MC AND CONDOMS (24 - 49 YEARS) 66
4.6. IEC WITH STI PREVENTION AND TREATMENT MESSAGES 67
4.7. VCT, MMC 68
4.8. MMC AND HIV/AIDS POLICY OPTIONS FOR CONSIDERATION 69
4.9. CONCLUSION 70

5. CHAPTER FIVE 73

5.1. RECOMMENDATIONS AND CONCLUSIONS 73
5.2 INTRODUCTION 73
5.3 RECOMMENDATIONS FOR KEY STAKEHOLDERS 73
5.4 THE CONTEXT OF POLICY IMPLEMENTATION AND CHALLENGES 76
5.5 THE COMMUNICATION PLAN 77
5.4 CONCLUSION 82

REFERENCES 85

APPENDIX I – SEARCH METHODS FOR OTHER SECTIONS 101

APPENDIX II THE MONITOR NEWSPAPER COMMENT 103

APPENDIX III UGANDA, HIV PREVALENCE BY REGION 105

APPENDIX IV OWNERSHPI OF HEALTH FACILITIES 107

APPENDIX V CONDOMS – CONFIDENCE BUILDING MEASURE 109

LIST OF TABLES

Table 1: Analysis of problem using the SWOT method................ 3
Table 2: Data base search 7
Table3: 2004-05 HIV prevalence in circumcised and uncircumcised men in selected tribes 16
Table 4: The Health infrastructure in Uganda 20
Table 5: Initiatives for HIV/AIDS prevention............................. 22
Table 6: SH related Policies / Practices at a glance...................... 30
Table 7: Advantages and disadvantages of Condoms in Uganda. 36
Table 8: Summary of the RCTs 45
Table 9: Advantages and disadvantages of MC.......................... 51
Table 10: Opportunities and Challenges of providing MC........... 60
Table 11: Criteria for policy appraisal and ranking..................... 63
Table 12: Policy issues for consideration in MC implementation in HIV/AIDS 69
Table 13: Recommendations for integrating MC intervention to for stakeholders... 73
Table 14: Challenges expected and how to overcome them......... 77

LIST OF FIGURES

Figure 1: The HIV/AIDS situational context in Uganda with MC28
Figure 2: Prospective relationships between policies, practices and MC 56
Figure 3: The model for policy Implementation.......................... 76

LIST OF PLATES

Plate 1: Sign post - Announcing a Health Centre II location in rural Uganda 19
Plate 2: One stop centre in Uganda with integrated range of reproductive health services.. 41
Plate 3: Campaign Communication post in Kampala, Uganda..... 59
Plate 4: A mobile HIV-testing site set up in a rural area of Uganda 69

LIST OF ACRONYMNS

ABC	Abstinence, Be faithful and Condom use
AB	Abstinence, Be faithful
ACP	Aids Control Programme
AIDS	Acquired Immunodeficiency syndrome
ANC	Antenatal Care
ART	Anti Retroviral Therapy
BBC	British Broadcasting Corporation
BMA	British Medical Association
BINGO's	Big Non-Governmental Organisations
BONGO's	Business Oriented Non-Governmental Organizations
CBOs	Community Based Organizations
CSW	Commercial Sex Workers
ESRC	Economic and Social Research Council
FB-PNFP	Faith Based Private Not for Profit
FGM	Female Genital Mutilation
FBOs	Faith Based Organisations
FP	Family Planning
HC	Health Centre
HIV	Human Immunodeficiency Virus
IEC	Information Education and Communication
LUL	Leeds University Library
MA	Master of Arts
MMC	Medical Male Circumcision
MC	Male Circumcision
MOH	Ministry of Health
MSM	Men who have Sex with Men
MPH	Master of Public Health
MTCT	Mother to Child Transmission
NGOs	Non Governmental Organizations
PEPFAR	President's Emergency Plan for AIDS Relief
PIT	Provider Initiated Testing
PIASCY	President's Initiative on AIDS Strategy Communicating to Young People
PMTCT	Prevention of Mother to Child Transmission

PNFP	Private Not For Profit
RCTs	Randomised Controlled Trials
STD	Sexually Transmitted Diseases
STI	Sexually Transmitted Infections
SH	Sexual Health
SWAP's	Sector Wide Approaches
SWOT	Strengths Weaknesses Opportunities and Threats
TB	Tuberculosis
UAC	Uganda Aids Commission
UCMB	Uganda Catholic Medical Bureau
UDHS	Uganda Demographic Health Survey
UMMB	Uganda Muslim Medical Bureau
UNAIDS	The Joint United Nations Programme on HIV/AIDS
UHSBS	Uganda HIV/AIDS Sero Behaviour Survey
UPMB	Uganda Protestant Medical Bureau
USAID	United States Agency for International Development
USA	United States of America
VCT	Voluntary Counselling and Testing
WHO	World Health Organization

GLOSSARY

Balanitis: Inflammation of the glans of the foreskin

Behaviour Dis-inhibition: Increased risk taking behaviour

Mucosa: Moist tissue that lines some organs like the penis

Phimosis: Condition where foreskin cannot be fully retracted

Risk compensation: Increased risk taking behaviour (behaviour dis-inhibition)

Zero grazing: Having sex with one sexual partner

EXECUTIVE SUMMARY

Dr Kevin De Cock[1] notes:

> "I hope we can move beyond the ABC debate — there will not be a single magic bullet for HIV prevention, it is more complicated than fixating on the alphabet, and we also need D and E. D for diagnosis (HIV testing) and E for everything else!"

Everything else is what is needed to achieve a sustained reduction in HIV infection in the world and more especially in Uganda with rates fluctuating between 5 – 10 % for more than 5 years. Reliance on one particular method(s) may expose sections of the population to greater risks. This could explain why for instance, married couples in Uganda (30 - 40 years) are increasingly getting infected with HIV/AIDS (UHSBS, 2006).

The aim of this dissertation is to explore HIV/AIDS and sexual health policies, and opportunities for inclusion of new interventions (like male circumcision) into the existing approaches, in order to reduce hetero- sexual HIV infection in men.

The objectives are to:

- Review the HIV/AIDS context in Uganda with emphasis on specific SH policies or practices and where other interventions can come in.
- Review available literature on MC and identify existing opportunities and challenges.
- Make an analysis of the medical, gender, ethical, social-economic and human rights dimension of MC as an HIV/AIDS prevention method.
- Suggest feasible recommendations for implementing successful HIV/AIDS and MC programmes in Uganda

For over twenty years, scientists have tried to establish through behavioural studies, the relationship between MC and HIV/AIDS. But it is the recent findings from RCTs conducted in South Africa, Kenya and Uganda that made a significant breakthrough.

In this discussion, I provide evidence from those and other studies; discussing them in the context of HIV/AIDS in Uganda. The basis for my argument is that, there are opportunities from research to enable policy makers adopt everything else at their disposal, including Medical Male Circumcision (MMC) to fight HIV/AIDS. This is despite some challenges!

The methods of analysis include literature searches and analysis, SWOT analysis, problem mind map, discussion of opinion, review of perspectives and a variety of tables for problem appraisal purposes.

Recommendations call for a gradual inclusion of MMC into the existing programmes while strengthening those strategies in place. The researcher concludes that, MMC as a programme can not succeed on its own. It needs the support of all stakeholders; the women, politicians, religious, funding agencies and men themselves.

[1] Dr Kevin De Cock is director of the HIV/Aids department of the World Health Organization.

General Introduction

Introduction

This chapter focuses on the justification of study, problem identification and analysis, the aims, objectives, methodology and the expected output. The stakeholders are also identified, as well as the role of the author.

Justification of the study

The increasing burden of HIV/AIDS in Uganda requires additional policy strategies into the existing prevention methods. These are needed to guide health professionals in adopting new programmes of reducing HIV infections in populations with unique social cultural contexts. Strong evidence now suggests that MC reduces HIV infection from HIV positive women to circumcised men by almost 60% (Baily, et al., 2006; Gray, et al., 2006; Auvert, et al., 2005). Several behavioural studies also consistently suggest lower HIV infection among circumcised men (Drain, et al., 2004; Reynolds, et al., 2004; Buve, 2002). This study builds on this evidence, to propose policy options for reducing HIV/AIDS infections, such as strengthening IEC in the existing prevention approaches.

The author does not in any way suggest that, MMC alone is a foolproof guarantee against HIV infection in men. Existing methods of prevention like ABC, STI prevention and treatment, proper IEC, ART and PMTCT are still recommended. This work only gives suggestions for widening the scope of HIV prevention in Uganda.

Problem Identification

The HIV/AIDS scourge is still a major problem in Uganda with adult prevalence (15 – 49 years) by the year 2003 estimated at 2.8 – 6.6% (WHO, 2005). Recent trends show that the infections and prevalence have gone up to 5.7 – 7.6% (UNAIDS 2007). The increased infections specifically noted among the 30 – 40 age group (UHSBS, 2006), suggests that the existing methods have not provided a sustained prevention against HIV infection for a group which was presumably well protected. These methods of HIV/AIDS prevention discussed elsewhere include the ABC strategy, STI prevention and treatment, IEC, ART and PMTCT. There has also been increased demand for MMC in Uganda (The BBC, 2007), which is a new form of intervention, but there is insufficient guidance on how it can be adopted as an HIV prevention approach in men. This demand for MC was driven by media highlights of findings mentioned in the justification above.

Problem Analysis

Problem analysis:

Table 1: Analysis of problem using the SWOT method

ANALYSIS	STRENGHTS	WEAKNESSES
Internal	**1.** Three randomised control trials (One conducted in Uganda) provide evidence that MC can reduce HIV infections in men by up to 60%. **2.** Practice mandatory in Muslim religious faith of Uganda which comprises 12.1% of total population. **3.** There has been increased demand for MC in Uganda. **4.** Uganda has experience in preventing HIV/AIDS infections, MC as an added opportunity can be used alongside other HIV /AIDS prevention measures. **5.** Some tribes in Uganda practice MC as a cultural obligation.	**1.** No proper MC policy in Uganda. **2.** Opposition from national reformist / Christian leadership (conservative ideologies and moralistic approaches). **3.** Relatively new phenomenon, no large-scale programme has been implemented in Uganda & elsewhere (except neo-natal MC in USA). **4.** No trained health workers in health centres to carry out MC. **5.** May be unpopular with the vast Ugandan Christian population (85.1%). **6.** Largely focussed on the male gender.
ANALYSIS	**OPPORTUNITIES**	**THREATS**
External	**1.** If implemented effectively, in long term, it can reduce infection in men, women and unborn children. **2.** Neonatal and adult surgery possible. **3.** Observational studies on	**1.** MC is not 100% effective; up to 40% infection can occur. **2.** Haemophilic (uncontrolled bleeding) threats may lead to death. **3.** Costs of

	MC and HIV/AIDS support MC to reduce infections. **4.** Medical operation can be performed once in a life time. **5.** MC reduces infections from STIs **6.** One off cost at operation – may not need other costs **7.** Support from International agencies like WHO, UNAIDS, USAID, PEPFAR and other international NGOs.	implementation could be high. **4.** Fears of risk compensation after MC (this can generate immoral behaviour). **5.** Infections may result if performed by unqualified staff. **6.** Pain when anesthesia is not used. **7.** Arguments that it reduces sexual pleasure in circumcised men. **8.** Can be questioned by human rights, especially neonatal MC. **9.** Likelihood of confusing MC with FGM. **10.** Threat to the condom market. It may be difficult to promote MC and condom use. **11.** Those who perform it as a cultural practice may reject it as compromising their culture eg. "Initiation" "manhood" rites.

Source: Author

Aim of the study

The aim of this study is to explore HIV/AIDS and sexual health policies and opportunities for inclusion of new interventions like

MMC into the existing approaches in order to reduce heterosexual HIV infection in men.

Objectives of the study

1) To review the HIV/AIDS context in Uganda with emphasis on specific SH policies and where other interventions can come in.
2) Review available literature on MC and identify existing opportunities and challenges.
3) Make an analysis of the medical, gender, ethical, social-economic and human rights dimension of MC as an HIV/AIDS prevention method.
4) Suggest feasible recommendations for implementing successful MC and HIV/AIDS prevention programmes in Uganda.

Methodology

The study area

The study focuses on the application of MC in Uganda's social, cultural and economic context. The situation is studied in consideration of existing HIV/AIDS prevention guidelines and practices. Experience is also drawn from relevant literature.

Sources of Data

Brain storming

The author began by brain storming the subject with fellow students on MA/MPH and colleagues on HIV/AIDS programmes in Uganda. The responses were helpful in giving me the initial perceptions held by different people.

Uganda government documents and the internet

I used the Uganda Government National Health policy documents, UHSBS, periodic HIV/AIDS country information, MOH Uganda, UNAIDS and WHO websites.

Alerts/Updates

a) Few Zetoc updates on MC with search string, "Male" & "Circumcision" & "HIV" in title, delivered by email between 24 February 2007 and 25 July 2007. In total 15 recently published papers were received. This probably indicates that there are not many new published papers at the time of this research.

b) Google alerts (with title "Male Circumcision HIV") were used to keep up to date with world opinion from National new papers, discussion papers and conference deliberations on MC. This provided me with added information on different opinions. More than 200 links to activities, blogs for and against MC, discussions and strategies were received. However, some information from the internet blogs was not quite reliable.

c) Follow up was also made on references from published works, and citations made from internet blogs received from alerts/updates in (b) above.

Web searches:

Searches were made from the Leeds University library, electronic data bases like Pubmed and the web of science (see table 2).

Table 2: Data base search

Data base	Keywords	Results	Refined
(i) LUL	Circumcision	5	2
(ii) The web of science	1. Circumcision	243	
	2.Circumcision.mp.or exp. circumcision	346	
	3.Circumcision, man, HIV infection	601607	
	Combined 1,2 and 3	243	243
(iii) Pubmed	1.Circumcision	3851	
	2. Male circumcision	2819	
	3. Neonatal circumcision	1086	
	4.cultur* male circumcision	269	
	Combined 3 and 2	968	968
	Combined 2 and HIV	17	17
	Combined 2 and HIV/AIDS	102	102
	Combined 3 and HIV/AIDS	09	09

The author manually browsed through the refined searches and reviewed the abstracts based on content and thematic relevance to the study. Peer reviewed journals published between 1992 and 2007 and those that met most criteria set by the systematic meta-analytic studies (discussed in 3.4.4) were considered. The search strategy for other sections is attached in Appendix I.

Design of evidence

I have presented three RCTs conducted in Africa. These are followed by two systematic reviews and meta-analysis studies on MC and heterosexual transmission of HIV in men from the Cochrane and the AIDS journal. Then results from behavioural studies on MC and HIV/AIDS are discussed. Finally, a selection of opinions from journals and internet sources are presented to guide the discussion.

Stake holders

This study will benefit a variety of stake holders like those involved in HIV interventions. These include political leaders, policy makers at the MOH, Providers of health and healthcare and the religious, UAC and ACP/STD of Uganda, and health professionals. This information will also be beneficial to national and international NGO's involved in HIV/AIDS prevention and researchers.

Scope

The scope here includes the context and policies in Uganda, sexual health practices, medical evidence, culture and human rights issues, opportunities and challenges that can be provided by MC.

Limitations

This study is limited by the fact that, adult MC is a practice which has never been implemented on a country level. The author has not come across literature to show successful adult MC implementation in large populations.

The output

Recommendations are made for prevention of HIV/AIDS considering MC and other interventions that have been in place. The opportunities and challenges that may arise in the implementation of MMC in a unique socio- economic environment are also identified. A communication plan is drawn as an action plan for stakeholders to start the HIV/AIDS and MMC integration process.

The role of the Author

I was previously involved in health education in Uganda. Some knowledge acquired from experience is included in this study.

During the course of this study, I have contributed to the ongoing policy discussion process for HIV/AIDS and MC, by writing to the Monitor Newspaper in Uganda (See Appendix II).

After the dissertation writing process, I will continue the discussion by getting involved in the communication process. I hope to share knowledge with interest groups, learn more and disseminate findings to stakeholders involved in HIV/AIDS prevention.

Outline of the dissertation

The overall structure of the dissertation is based on elements of policy analysis proposed in a framework by Collins, (2005), which involves defining context, stating problem, searching for evidence, considering different policy options, projecting outcomes, criteria for evaluation, weighing outcome and making a decision.

The first part of the dissertation is the introduction. It has the justification, problem, aim, objectives, methodology, the scope, limitations, role of the author and outline of the study.

Chapter one gives the background to the HIV/AIDS problem in Uganda. The chapter identifies the HIV prevalence in Uganda, the risk factors involved, initiatives and barriers.
In chapter two, a brief description is made of specific HIV/AIDS policies like the ABC, STI, IEC, VCT and mention of the ART and PMTCT interventions.

Chapter three discusses opportunities like its acceptability from women, international bodies and neo-natal MC. I also provide opinions about MC in other social settings. Challenges are discussed by looking at costs, consent and human rights issues.

In chapter four, the policy options are described and appraised, after which a strategy is identified. The final chapter gives the recommendations, communication plan and the final conclusion.

Conclusion

This chapter has provided the justification for widening the scope of HIV/AIDS interventions forms in Uganda due to increasing infections from HIV/AIDS. Despite the strengths identified that MC reduces HIV infection in circumcised men, there are still many threats seen from the SWOT analysis (Table 1). The methodology depicts the variety of information sources consulted. This chapter has also identified the stakeholders and others to benefit from the study. The next chapter is an exploration of the background context and the factors predisposing people to HIV/AIDS in Uganda.

1. CHAPTER ONE

1.1. Introduction

The preceding chapter has identified the problem and considered the need for this study. This chapter gives some background information on Uganda and the factors that have affected the current HIV/AIDS situation. This is helpful in understanding how further changes to policies affecting HIV/AIDS may be influenced by some of aspects mentioned here.

1.2. General Demographic data

Uganda, located in Sub Saharan Africa, has a population of approximately 28 million people with about 38% living below the national poverty line of US$ 300 p.a. Per capita income is US$ 338 (2004/2005). The average life expectancy (2005) was 49.5 (males 48.0; females 51.0). Mortality before the age of five is 136 per 1000. The population growth rate is estimated at 3.3% (WHO, 2005). Maternal mortality is 527 per 100,000 (UDHS, 2001).

1.3. HIV/AIDS in Uganda

Uganda has now battled HIV/AIDS for more than 20 years and HIV/AIDS is still one of the greatest challenges with an estimated 1,000,000 people being HIV positive. About 60,000 out of 114,000 of those clinically eligible for ART by the end of the year 2005 are able to access therapy (WHO, 2005).

According to the 2004- 2005 survey, the prevalence has stabilised at 5 - 10% in urban areas and below 5% in the rural areas. Uganda has made significant gains in Africa in reducing HIV prevalence from 18% in 1992 to 6.4 in 2005. But hetero-sexual transmissions still accounts for 76% of the new infections, where CSWs account for 21%, casual sex 14% and infections within marriage 42%; MTCT accounts for between 22- 25%. The antenatal HIV sero-prevalence in urban areas was between 5.4 and 12.5 percent. While for sites located in the semi-urban and rural areas, it ranged from 1.3 to 7.9 percent. A comparison drawn from the results suggests that the regional distribution of the level of antenatal HIV sero-prevalence from the sentinel surveillance system is similar to that observed in the population-based survey (UHSBS, 2006). The details are indicated on the Map of Uganda in Appendix III.

There is a higher risk of HIV infections among urban residents, which is 10% compared to 6% among rural residents. Prevalence among urban women is 13% compared with 7% for rural women.

Prevalence among urban men is 7% compared with 5% for rural men. Central, Kampala (the capital) and North Central regions all have rates of infection above 8%. Regions with low HIV prevalence are West Nile (2%) and Northeast (4%). Women have a higher prevalence of HIV infection than men in all regions (ŬHSBS, 2006).

1.4. Determinants and consequences

There are several factors affecting the spread and increase of HIV/AIDS in Uganda. Some of the factors are cultural, religious, economic and political.

1.4.1. Cultural practices and attitudes

HIV infections vary from tribe to tribe, and are affected by some cultural practices, like beliefs (that AIDS is caused by witchcraft), and customary or religious practices like MC. For instance, MC is performed as a cultural obligation for tribes in the Bududa, Manafwa, Mbale and Sironko, Kasese and Bundibugyo Districts of Uganda (Authors observation). In table 3 below, HIV/AIDS prevalence is noted to be different in tribes and geographic locations of circumcising and non-circumcising tribes of Uganda.

Table 3: 2004-05 HIV prevalence in circumcised and uncircumcised men in selected tribes

Ethnicity	Circumcised men 15-49		Uncircumcised men 15-49	
	% HIV positive	**Number**	**% HIV positive**	**Number**
Baganda	**3.6**	**402**	**6.7**	903
Banyankore	**2.6**	**68**	**6.1**	707
Iteso	**(6.8)**	**35**	**4.5**	58
Lugbara / Madi	**2.8**	**213**	**1.9**	349
Basoga	**2.7**	**236**	**7.2**	449
Langi	*	**8**	**7.2**	424
Bakiga	**(10.4)**	**42**	**3.6**	495
Karimojong	*	**11**	**1.2**	177
Acholi	*	**18**	**6.5**	325
Bagisu / Sabiny	**4.3**	**359**	**0.0**	91
Alur / Jopadhola	**6.0**	**73**	**3.9**	339
Banyara	**(7.0)**	**38**	**6.8**	209
Batoro	**(7.8)**	**44**	**14.3**	153
All others	1.8	308	4.0	526

Note: Totals include some cases with missing information. Numbers in parentheses are based on 25-49 unweighted cases; an asterisk refers to a figure based on fewer than 25 cases that has been suppressed.
Source: UHSBS, (2006).

The above results from selected tribes show a higher HIV prevalence among uncircumcised men than in the circumcised men. It is however worrying to note a higher HIV prevalence among Bagishu/Sabiny (4.3%) who practice culturally performed MC, compared to circumcised men in Buganda (3.6%). It is important to establish whether culturally performed MC and its rural location of Bagisu/Sabiny has disadvantaged it in comparison to Buganda's urban location.

1.4.2. Long term impact of HIV/AIDS

HIV/AIDS has for long been a major cause of morbidity and mortality in Uganda with devastating effects. The disease has hit the country severely, with infection having at one time hit up to 30% and life has been affected in different ways. The major observable effects have been the number of orphans due to HIV/AIDS. According to the Uganda government (2007), the estimated number of orphans due to AIDS is 890,000 (45.6%) of all orphans. This has also affected the socio-economic development of the country through loss of the productive manpower. The causes for this continued increase in the problem are varied.

1.4.3. Role of religious bodies in Health

The religious organisations, recognised as FB- PNFP in Uganda are very influential in health and healthcare delivery and even HIV/AIDS prevention. They operate under umbrella organisations like the UCMB, UPMB and the UMMB representing 78% of the

509 PNFP health units. These bureaus own a large health infrastructure base of hospitals and health centres. For instance, they own 42 out of the 98 hospitals in Uganda and 509 (24%) of the 2158 lower level units which are predominantly located in rural areas. In addition, they provide health services and train health workers. They also operate 20 health training schools out of the 48 in the country (The republic of Uganda, 2003).

1.4.4. Political organisation and HIV/AIDS

The UAC is in charge of aspects of HIV/AIDS policy formulation, planning implementation and identifying barriers of programmes related to HIV/AIDS. The decentralised districts of Uganda are required to have a mechanism that addresses specific HIV/AIDS issues. These include coordination, a development plan, and support for CBOs which implement HIV/AIDS issues (The Republic of Uganda, 2006b). Such a mechanism is supposed to be helpful in promoting HIV/AIDS interventions which need the involvement of different stakeholders. However, the capacity of local governments may still be very weak because of lack of funding, corruption and different priorities of local government development (Jeppsson, 2001).

1.4.5. The Health infrastructure

The description of health facilities' structure in Table 4 below shows the capabilities which certain health centres have in the facilitation of specific health care roles. From the structure, it is evident that HC IV which is normally situated at the health sub districts is the one that has the infrastructure for surgeries. This is because of the resources mentioned. But the distribution of HC IV's in Uganda still shows a general inadequacy as can be noted in their distribution throughout the country (see Appendix IV).

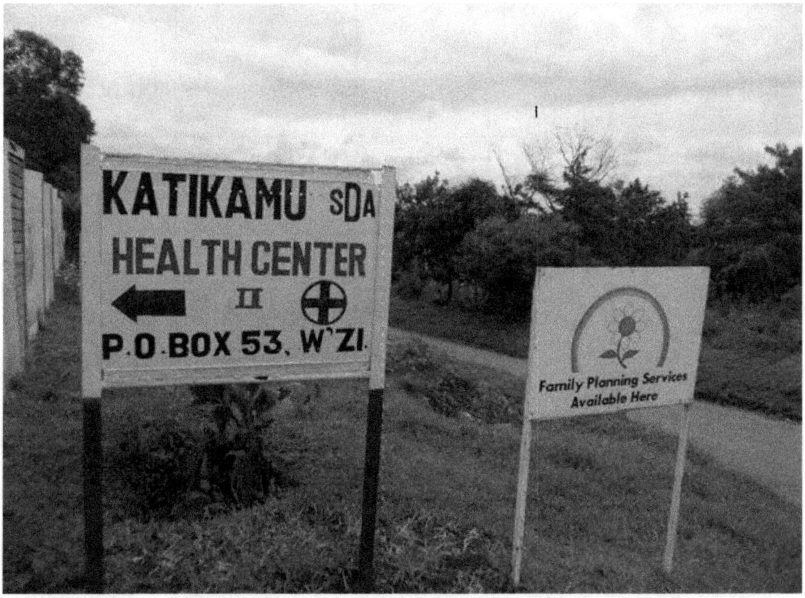

Plate 1: Sign post - Announcing a Health Centre II location in rural Uganda (Source: author)

Table 4: The Health infrastructure in Uganda

Facility	Grad / type	Location	Services	Staff
Health Centre	II	Parish level	Outpatient care, ANC, immunisation and outreach	1 enrolled nurse, 1 enrolled midwife and 2 nursing assistants (or comprehensive nurse).
Health Centre	III	Sub county	All services in HC II plus inpatient care and environmental health	1 clinical officer, 1 enrolled nurse, 2 enrolled midwives and 1 nursing assistant, 1 health assistant, 1 laboratory assistant and a Records Officer
Health Centre	IV	Sub district	All services at HC III, surgery, supervises the lower units HC IIs and IIIs, collects and analyses health data and plans for the health sub-district	1 medical officer, 2 clinical officers, registered midwife, enrolled nurse, enrolled midwife, comprehensive nurse, 2 nursing assistants, laboratory technician, laboratory assistant,

				health inspector, dispenser, public health dental assistant, Anaesthetic Officer, one Asstt Health Educator, one Records Assit, 1Accounts Assit, 2 support staff
Hospitals (Government and Non Government)	National referral / regional referral, district & rural hospitals	Cities, regional towns, districts rural hospitals	Referral and Specialists limited fields	Teaching, general doctors

Source: Uganda Government (2007a)

1.4.6. Human resources for health

The human resource situation for health is also in a poor state. There is short supply of mid – level cadres like clinical officers and public health nurses. There is a slow and inadequate responsiveness of the training system to the planned requirements. In-service as nationally planned, has not been feasible. Selection of trainees favours candidates from the central region and larger hospitals hence disadvantage the rural and remote. This training of human resource is also affected by inadequate budgets, equipment and lack of accommodation facilities. There are poor attitudes and discipline; poor motivation and supervision (The Republic of Uganda, 2006b).

From this description of human resource, it can be seen that the current system is still constrained. Such a force cannot meet the day to day health and health care needs of the population. These challenges are also more likely to be faced when the system adopts new strategies to expand on the provision of services.

1.4.7. Sources of funding for HIV/AIDS

The major source of funding for HIV/AIDS in Uganda is the Global Fund, having so far disbursed 139,562, 348 US dollars for round 1 to round 6 to tackle HIV/AIDS, malaria and TB (Global Fund, 2007). Uganda's expenditure on HIV/AIDS and TB is still below the 15% minimum target recommended in the Abuja declaration by African Heads of state to allocate to these diseases (WHO, 2005a).

1.5. Current HIV/AIDS initiatives

In response to HIV/AIDS, there are a number of initiatives that are in place to address the problem as summarised in the following table.

Table 5: Initiatives for HIV/AIDS prevention

Initiative	Target group	Present	challenge
ART	All HIV positive persons	Only about 65,000 access ARTs out of	People have not wholly responded to

		150,000 (50%).	ART because of stigmatization fears.
Abstinence /faithful	Young people 15 – 19 years and married couples	Abstinence and faithfulness partially effective	It is very difficult to enforce or enhance abstinence and faithfulness.
Condoms	High risk Sexually active groups	Inconsistent condom supply	Over reliance of abstinence and conflicting messages.
STIs	Men and women 15 – 49 years	STI prevalence noted among youths.	Poor response to STI treatment
PMTCT	HIV positive mothers (Even HIV negative are targeted)	Less than 10% of women targeted for PMTCT in 2005	Low coverage, only about 10% of pregnant women covered.
IEC	All	Not well coordinated	Gets weakened sometimes / not consistent
VCT	Men and women 15-19 years	Poor response, especially for men	Not spread out

Source: Author

The above table shows that the initiatives for HIV/AIDS prevention in place are still insufficient. Further weaknesses and barriers to some of these methods are discussed in the next chapter.

1.6. Religious barriers to HIV/AIDS programme

There are a number of barriers to the existing interventions for reducing HIV infections in Uganda. One of these is the Catholic

Church's strong opposition to the use of condoms. This Church worldwide is still opposed to the use of any form of contraceptives for birth control and any sexual health intervention based on scientific discovery. In a message presented at the XIV International AIDS conference entitled, "Belated, but powerful" (2002), the church recognised that she would "situate HIV/AIDS in the wider context of the gospel understanding of and a values-based approach…" As such they encourage abstinence and being faithful as a major component of their strategy in HIV prevention messages. This view is widely supported by the reformist Christians churches in Uganda. Their argument is that, sexual health interventions that do not promote abstinence alone encourage careless sexual lifestyles. This is the reason why condoms have been unpopular with some Christians in Uganda (Authors observation).

1.7. Political barriers

Uganda's success story of reducing HIV/AIDS has also come as a result of a combined effort of the president of Uganda. There are several presidential initiatives that target specific groups like the PIASCY and the First lady of Uganda's youth initiatives. But their insistences on Abstinence and virginity campaigns have drawn a lot of criticisms from international human rights activists; the policy shift is seen as an influence from the USA government (Human Rights watch, 2005). The president of Uganda was also quoted to have told a students' medical convention at Makerere

University that MC was not a solution to HIV/AIDS (The New Vision, 2006).

1.8. Corruption

This has also been a major hindrance to the proper implementation of HIV/AIDS programmes in Uganda. The Global Fund suspended Uganda's allocations of funds to fight AIDS, Tuberculosis and malaria to a tune of $201 million due to corruption (Eaton, 2005)). This was an unfortunate development because it would lead to death of people who were on treatment like ART and increase resistance of diseases like T.B to drug treatment (Eaton, 2005a).

1.9. Conclusion

From the above descriptions, it is evident that the HIV/AIDS context in Uganda is riddled with several problems which not only predispose people to HIV/ADS, but also may increase the epidemic. Noted are issues of culture, religion, politics, corruption, the infrastructure and funding for the existing interventions. In the next chapter, I identify specific HIV/AIDS sexual health policies in Uganda; and areas where other forms of intervention may come in to improve the situation.

2. CHAPTER TWO

2.1 HIV/AIDS, Sexual Health policies and MC

2.2 Introduction

The preceding chapter has made some explanation of the HIV/AIDS environment and the factors that predispose people to HIV/AIDS in Uganda. In here, I establish whether existing interventions have been effective in addressing the problem. In so doing, I try to identify the policies in place, what they have achieved and some shortcomings. Figure 1 below depicts such relations, in light of the context already described.

Figure 1: The HIV/AIDS situational context in Uganda with MC

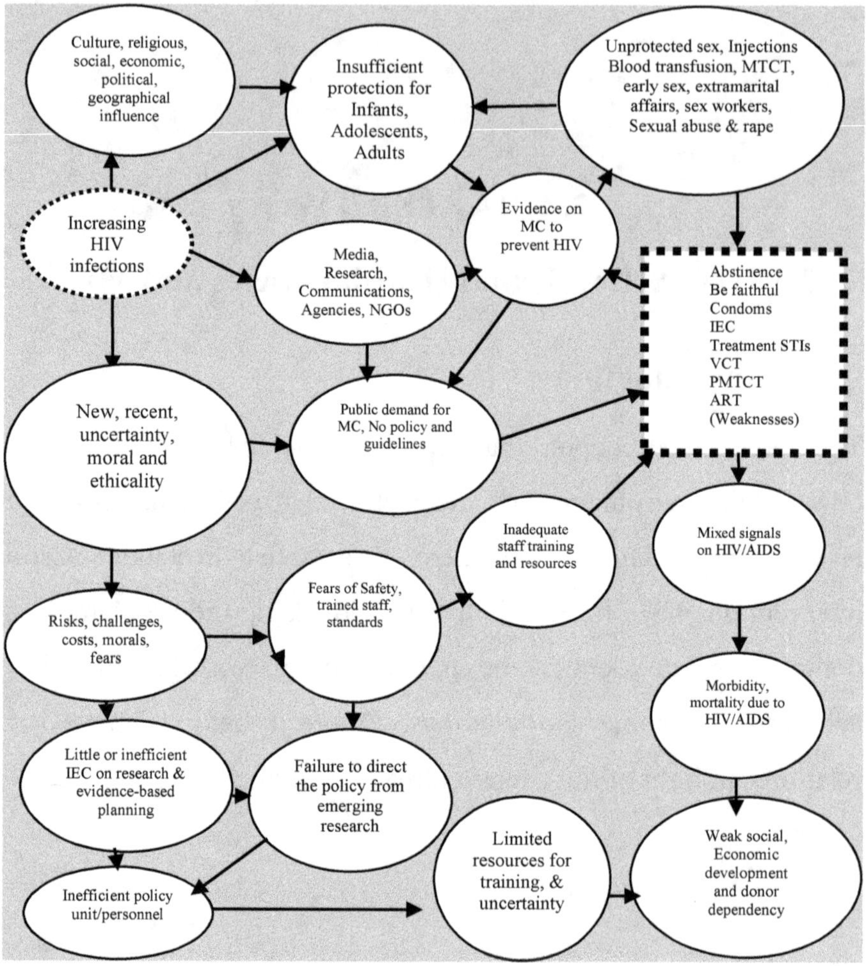

Source: Author

The figure above shows that the increasing HIV infections are determined by cultural, economic, religious, political factors. These have affected all age groups through unprotected sex, injections, blood transfusion, MTCT, early sex, extramarital affairs, CSW, Sexual abuse and rape.

2.3 Definition of Policy

In the course of this discussion, I have adopted Walt, (1994)'s definition of health policy, which,

> Embraces courses of action that affect the set of institutions, organizations, services and funding arrangements of the health care system. It goes beyond health services, however, and includes actions or intended actions by public, private and voluntary organizations that have impact on health. (p41).

This definition is preferred because; it looks at policy from a wider socio- economic perspective. It also involves more institutions, organizations or individuals referred to as actors. This will help me to reflect on what has been in place, in an effort to do a simple 'analysis of policy,' in order to project policy options for the future, known as, 'analysis for policy' (Parson, 1995).

2.4 Background to Uganda's HIV/AIDS policy

According to the Uganda National Health policy (1999p11), STIs/HIV/AIDS would best be managed through:

> A program of intense IEC aimed at promoting responsible sexual and reproductive behaviour; sexual and reproductive counselling; HIV counselling and testing; wide use of condoms; prompt treatment of STIs; universal blood safety; reduction of mother to child transmission; palliative care; promotion of community involvement in the care of patients with AIDS and mitigation of the socio- economic impact of the epidemic.

The above policy descriptions focus on programs that are a key in HIV/AIDS prevention but also need to emphasize STI prevention.

For this study, I have chosen to concentrate on policy guidelines for primary HIV/AIDS prevention, mainly the ABC, STIs, VCT and IEC. These policy practices have been selected because they target HIV negative men. The RCTs (See 3.4.1), also investigated the primary efficacy of MC on participants who were HIV negative (Baily, *et al.,* 2006; Gray, *et al.,* 2006; Auvert, *et al.*, 2005). For that reason, programmes like PMTCT and ART have not been extensively reviewed. On the other hand, blood safety accounts for 2% of HIV infections in Uganda (Okware, 2004), but it is beyond the scope of this study. Table 5 below, gives a summary of some sexual health policies in Uganda. They are afterwards discussed to show some gaps and barriers. It is important to note that, the policies and practices below would be judged as good if they are accessible to all, effective and acceptable to the rich, poor, women and men.

Table 6: SH related Policies / Practices at a glance

Aspect of Policy/practice	Description of policy	Target	Process	Expected output
Abstinence	Abstinence - Avoid any sexual activities that cause HIV transmission.	Young people 14 – 18 years	communication by NGOs, Government, CBOs,FBOs	Reporting of virginity increase, delayed first sexual debut

Faithfulness	Be faithful – Sexual intercourse only with mutually faithful uninfected partner	- Married persons	Communication by NGOs, Government, CBOs, FBOs	Reduced number of non- regular partners for married men and women, commitment to marriage.
Condoms*	Adoption of correct and consistent use of condoms backed by appropriate education	- All Persons involved in high risk sexual behaviour - HIV positive and discordant couples - Couples in serial monogamy	- Free distribution of condoms through public sector - Social marketing of condoms	More correct and consistent use of condoms, reduced STI and HIV
STIs	Early, prompt and proper treatment of STIs, syndromic management of STIs	- men, women, never married, currently married, formerly married	- Campaigns to prevent STIs, training health workers at all levels in STI care and investment in purchase of drugs.	Reduced self-reporting of STIs and reduced diagnosis of STI in STI clinics

VCT	Provision of VCT services by health workers and counsellors appropriately to all people in order to help bring about positive behaviour change	Clients in need of TB, FP, STD, ART, PMTCT and similar services	Awareness of existence of VCT services, counselling, testing, post test counselling and post test care.	Increased utilisation of VCT facilities, increased number of persons testing for HIV
IEC	Unlimited access to information using available media to reach all categories of the population	All	- Radio, drama, T.V and leaflets, awareness	Access to IEC facilities and behaviour change responses due to IEC

*Condoms here mainly refer to male condoms (See 3.4.8)
Source: Author with ideas from; Okware, et al., (2005)

2.5 The behavioural Approach

There have been combined efforts that advocate for several approaches to reduce infection from HIV and also mitigate severity of HIV/AIDS in Uganda. The multi- methodical approach, has among others proposed the abstinence, faithfulness and condom use, commonly known as the ABC strategy. Much as this approach has played a positive role, it has got some challenges as noted in the following literature.

2.5.1 Abstinence

Abstinence involves primary abstinence, where young persons delay their first sexual activity and secondary abstinence, where a person stops sex after first initiation (Okware, *et al.,* 2005). Abstinence programmes in Uganda have mainly focussed on young people being given information for better sexual behaviour. It encourages better peer interaction and decision making within a good education system, which implements a recommended health curriculum (Shue, *et al.,* 1999).

There has been increased reliance on abstinence advocated for the young persons (14 – 19 years) in Uganda towards reducing infection. Positive trends have been realised, with age of first sexual initiations reducing to 16% in men (15 – 19 years) and 12% in women (15 – 19 years) (UHSBS, 2006). But abstinence, only gives a protective value to the young people in delayed age of first sexual debut and increased virginity, lasting up to the age of 19 years (Okware, *et al.,* 2005).

It should also be noted that, HIV reduction in Uganda has arisen out of a combination of factors, not just abstinence (Green, *et al.,* 2006). This argument is supported by Singh (2003.p129) that:

> When all changes in sexual behaviour are taken into consideration, the effect of increased abstinence on the overall level of sexual exposure to risk of HIV is moderated

From their observations, abstinence programmes need to be repackaged with a better focus. Not only have abstinence programmes undermined condom benefits, they are also taught to the sexually active people. Such factors have unfortunately made abstinence fail to work even among the born again Christian youths considered religious in Uganda (Sadgrove, 2007).

2.5.2 Faithfulness

Being faithful, also known as zero grazing is also a moral, integrity, ethical approach of responding to HIV/AIDS, just like abstinence. Faithfulness has also played a significant role in bringing down the prevalence of HIV/AIDS in Uganda, because people are now faithful by having sex with fewer partners (Green, *et al.,* 2006; Okware, *et al*., 2005). But in marriage where it is promoted in Uganda, several concerns may come up. For example, married partners cannot guarantee commitment of each others' safety from HIV infection. Neither can it work in cultures where women are socialized to obey men or in abusive relationships (Mpagi, 2005). Faithfulness is also difficult to ascertain in polygamous relationships or marriages.

2.5.3 Condoms

There is sufficient evidence to suggest that condoms give a high degree of protection against STIs and HIV (Rietmeijer, *et al.,* 1988). In Uganda, this has been backed by the promotion of condoms in a policy of open and efficient distribution and responsible use of male and female condoms, with appropriate education (The Republic of Uganda, 2004). There has also been renewed support for condoms in Uganda from the technical level to energise condom use as a confidence building measure, to increase public faith in condoms (see Appendix V). This follows problems of inconsistent supply, quality, administration and controversies that have characterised the condom debate in Uganda in the past three years (Wakabi, 2006; Bass, 2005). As already noted (in section 1.3.4), there have been negative influences to the condom use by sections of revivalist movements from the USA. Huge funds have been invested to change messages in schools from condom use, to abstinence, which has had a negative effect on condom use (Human Rights watch, 2005).

But, low use of condoms is still associated with beliefs, attitudes, misconceptions or biases among the community. In sections of African communities, people perceive condoms as mainly family planning kits to prevent pregnancies (Maharaj, 2006). Even in societies where polygamy is a norm and premarital relationships for men is acceptable, men do not use them, despite knowing their protective benefits against HIV (Oyedirani, 2003). This kind of thinking continues to place the condom at a disadvantaged position in the fight against HIV/AIDS.

Such attitudes associated with condom use need to be addressed through extensive IEC. For instance, existing attitudes which state that you cannot use a condom with a trusted partner or the one you love, and that condom sex is not pleasurable (Manuel, 2005, Muhwava, 2004), are discouraging. These attitudes may however not be widespread in Uganda where there has been widespread IEC in the media about HIV/AIDS (Green, *et al*., 2006).

Available literature suggests that, in some cases, high risk sexually active groups have been noted to incorrectly use condoms, which lead to condoms breaking during sex (Mukenge,*et al*., 2005). This can be very dangerous and can only encourage the spread of HIV.

On the whole, Okware, *et al.,* (2005) acknowledge the need of condoms for those who are HIV positive, the discordant couples living together, the sex workers, those in short term relationships and for the prevention of STIs.

In table 7 below, the advantages and disadvantages of condoms are identified.

Table 7: Advantages and disadvantages of Condoms in Uganda

Advantages	Disadvantage
Give significant protection against STD's and HIV.	Requires very consistent and careful use
Very effective when used correctly and consistently	Has tendency of encouraging sexual recklessness
No side effects, allergies to latex not largely reported	Can be quite expensive for some
No prescription required, simple instructions for use	Inconsistent supply in Uganda in the past
Generally affordable	Pro- Abstinence and faithfulness

	campaigners castigate it
Available in village local shops	Perceived as FP tool
Distributed free in public health facilities	Attitudes that condoms reduce sexual pleasure

Source: Author

The table above shows that, condoms provide a significant protection against STIs and HIV though with some disadvantages.

2.6 STIs

STIs are still a significant health problem in Uganda. Up to 33% of women (20 – 39 yrs) and 21% of men (25 -49 yrs) sexually active have reported having symptoms of STIs infections (UHSBS, 2006). There is higher STIs infection in women groups compared to men. STIs still account for about 20% of the adult outpatient consultation in public health facilities (Uganda government, 2003a). There is poor response to treatment of STIs because of stigmatization, prejudices and delayed response to treatment. The situation is aggravated by the poor management of STIs in Uganda's formal and informal health facilities (Jacobs, *et al.*,2003).

A recent survey in Uganda showed that, circumcised men were less likely to report having had an STI infection. Lower HIV prevalence was also noted in circumcised men than the circumcised (UHSBS, 2006). These findings confirm that STIs facilitate the transmission of HIV (Reynolds, *et al.,* 2006; Ofarrell,

1999). STIs have also been identified as a risk factor as well as a symptom of HIV infection (Sserwadda, *et al.*, 2003).

The above findings are helpful insights for widening the scope of methods available for an effective STI prevention and treatment, which may consequently lead to reduced HIV infections.

2.7 VCT services

The global trend towards VCT is still very low. Only about 12% of those who want to be tested are able to do so. About 0.4% of adults in 2005 in the 15 – 49 years age bracket in low and middle income countries received HIV tests through routine counselling and testing. Sub Saharan Africa, noted with the highest utilization of testing achieved 2.2% (WHO, 2006).

The use of VCT services in Africa is low and also largely captures women who attend ANC services. Even in such situations, the overall acceptance of VCT is hindered by stigmatization of the HIV infected people (Magoni, *et al.,* 2007; Okonkwo, *et al,* 2007). The above situations make it difficult for people to benefit from VCT services, which are an opportunity to benefit from an intervention of reducing HIV infection.

The cost of VCT services being high may also be a hindrance if it is not provided free of charge. For example, in countries with limited resources, provision of wide scale VCT are an enormous challenge because such costs can only decline with an expanded scale of VCTs (McConnel, *et al.*, 2005). A VCT venture would be very cost effective in averting the cost of HIV infection by up to $2000 (Sweat, *et al.,* 2000). Such a measure, if provided with an intervention like condom use would blend well in a wide comprehensive HIV reduction strategy, which is suggested by the World Health Organization in the universal access for all (WHO, 2006).

It should be noted however that, VCT has not been a success story all through. In some places where VCT is free and accessible in rural areas, minimal impact has been realised on reducing risk behaviour and incidence of HIV infection (Matovu, *et al.*, 2005). Low uptake of VCT services have also been noted in places where costs have been subsidised (Wolff, *et al.*, 2005). Not only would there be need to put up VCT services for homes where there are no service constraints and social barriers (Matovu, *et al.*, 2002), but also, a further exploration on why men do not utilise VCT services would help to improve this process.

From the above discussion, it should be recognised that, improving VCT access and acceptance for the population in the rural and urban areas is crucial. These people would benefit from existing interventions and new ones being proposed.

2.8 IEC

An effective IEC is essential in addressing issues of public health benefit. Better IEC were critical in reducing the level of HIV infection in Uganda (Stoneburner & Low-Beer, 2004). But sometimes, IEC channels have not been effectively used to put across HIV/AIDS related messages (Mitchell, *et al.,* 2001). For all interventions aimed at reducing the high prevalence of HIV and AIDS, there is need for a proper IEC to enhance understanding of messages among people in the rural and urban areas; especially among the illiterate communities.

2.9 ART and PMTCT

ART and PMTCT form an integral part of the HIV/AIDS prevention package which has not been extensively discussed in this study. These are secondary interventions that I consider as very important. They are part of the wider strategy that can be effectively promoted through VCT, IEC to complement existing methods of HIV/AIDS prevention. I recognise that, it is important to promote ART and PMCTC. This would be striving towards universal access for all, as recommended by the World Health Organization (WHO, 2006).

2.10 Conclusion

In this chapter, I have discussed the HIV/AIDS intervention policies in Uganda. From the reviews of what exists, the ABC strategy is still helpful, but has not been very successful. The response of the people in the use of condoms and even treatment of STIs is low. Infections with STIs are noted to increase the transmission of HIV but MC is also identified as reducing STI infections. There is also evidence that response to VCT is low and sometimes IEC messages are not well managed. Mention is made of ART and PMTCT. It is in these gaps and barriers noted that other forms of interventions may be integrated to address the problem. In the next chapter, a review of MC as an intervention method in HIV/AIDS prevention is made, by identifying the opportunities and challenges.

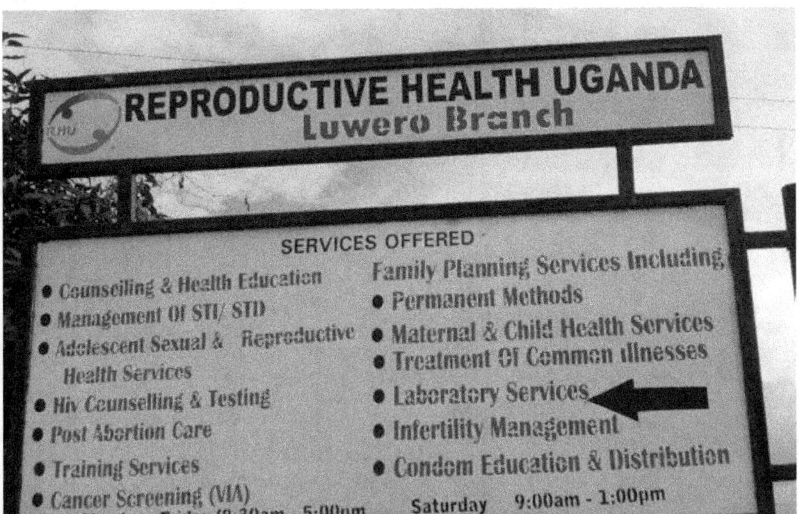

Plate 2: One stop centre in Uganda with integrated range of reproductive health services
(Source: author)

3. CHAPTER THREE

3.1 Opportunities and Challenges of MC

3.2 Introduction

The preceding chapter has endeavoured to highlight the HIV/AIDS policy context in Uganda, looking at a selection of some policies and practices. The author has also demonstrated that, the approaches followed have some weaknesses. This is where MC could come in to complement those interventions in place. In this chapter, an attempt is made to define and assess the evidence that MC reduces HIV infection in circumcised men. The challenges and opportunities offered by MMC are also identified.

3.3 What is MC?

MC is the surgical removal of the tissue covering the head of the penis (UNAIDS, 2007). For long, MC has borne a variety of associations; as a distinguishing priestly class, initiation of boys into the community of men, signal of God's chosen people and also marking the circumcised as superior in health (Gollaher, 1999). The practice of MMC can be performed by qualified medical personnel and the operation can last up to 30 minutes. Such a procedure has also been proved to work in the context of a resources limited environment that can be applied in poor countries (Krieger, 2005).

3.4 Opportunities provided by MC

MC provides numerous opportunities as a surgical practice that prevents infection from HIV in men. Below, an endeavour is made to discuss the opportunities which are available as evidence to that effect:

3.4.1 The medical trials on MC

The evidence from 3 RCTs (Baily, *et al.,* 2006; Gray, *et al.,* 2006; Auvert, *et al.,* 2005) provide consistent data, which can be relied on in making decisions. In calling for this evidence based health policy, Frammer and Rychetnik (2003), note among other things that, it is important to know how effective interventions are, and know that the benefits of an intervention outweigh any harmful effects. The evidence on MC below can be a basis for policies of primary public health interventions, in reducing HIV infection in men.

The trials below all consistently agree that, MC reduces the risks of men acquiring HIV by more than 50% of cases. In table 8, an assessment is made of the strengths and weaknesses of this evidence and its relevance thereafter.

Table 8: Summary of the RCTs

Setting and study objective			Design	Findings
South Africa (Orange farm)	Determine impact of MC on the acquisition of HIV by young men and assess the role of behavioural factors associated with HIV sero-status to explain its impact		Semi urban based population. **Cases**: Only data from uncircumcised males aged 18-24 years whose sero-status is negative was analysed. MC was also provided to HIV positive participants. **Intervention**: Immediate MC within a week of randomisation **Control**: Delayed MC operation	There were 20 participants who acquired HIV in the intervention group, odds ratio 0.85 (0.55-1.32) and 49 participants in the control group acquired HIV odds ratio 2.1 (1.6 – 2.8). MC protection of up to 60% During a period of 21 months, circumcised men prevented infection by six out of ten potential infections. Risky sexual behaviour increased slightly in intervention group (more sexual contacts)
Uganda (Rakai)	Investigate the effect of male circumcision on HIV incidence in men		Rural community based treatment groups generated in blocks of 20 in different sections of the population.	A significant reduction of HIV among circumcised men with efficacy rate of 51% compared to uncircumcised

			Cases: Uncircumcised HIV negative persons 15- 49 years with status confirmed at screening **Intervention:** MC surgery provided within two weeks of enrolment **Control:** Delayed MC operation	men. Noted MC reduction of HIV in men without behavioural dis-inhibition
Kenya (Kisumu)	Determine whether MC has a protective effect against HIV infection and to assess safety and changes in sexual behaviour related to intervention		Ethnic based urban study in population that does not normally circumcise was recruited. **Cases**: Uncircumcised HIV negative persons, 18 – 24 years who are sexually active. **Intervention**: MC surgery provided the same day or shortly thereafter. **Control**: Delayed MC until the end of study	There were 22 men who became HIV positive among the circumcised group (incidence 2.1%) and 47 in the uncircumcised group (incidence 4.2%). MC protection of up to 53%. There was noted little difference in circumcised and uncircumcised men's change in sexual behaviour.

Source: Author, with notes from (Baily, *et al* 2006; Gray, *et al.,* 2006; Auvert, *et al.,* 2005)

3.4.2 Challenges noted from RCTs

From the South African study, risky sexual behaviour increased slightly in the intervention group. The above RCTs were also conducted in a "healthcare paradise" environment unavailable in rural African settings. It is also noted that, participants were encouraged and provided with a great opportunity to use condoms whose effect is not properly stated (*Who used more condoms? the circumcised or uncircumcised?).* This may have reduced infections in circumcised men very significantly. The strength of the supportive services provided like STI treatment, ART, VCT did play a huge role. On the psychology level, it is possible that fear characterised men after MC who deliberately delayed their sexual activity after MC, in order not to take chances of acquiring HIV.

These studies have no major implications for neonatal MC. They do not address possible direct reductions of infection in women or MSM. They also do not address long term effectiveness of MC on HIV infection in hetero sexual men. The population can still be considered small, which may provide hardships of implementing MC in a larger population.

3.4.3 Policy Implications

It can be noted from the studies that IEC is very crucial in promoting MC. If MC should be an intervention considered in Uganda's setting, it will require huge investments in training of personnel, acquisition of facilities and equipment for the operation.

The above findings also provide key specific messages that need to be considered in drawing up plans for implementing any MC related intervention in a wider population:

- The overall need for VCT services in places that are inaccessible.
- Provision of condoms to people with high risk sexual behaviour.
- An effective IEC that incorporates ABC messages for the young people 14- 18 years.
- The need to emphasise that MC is not fool-proof protection against HIV infection
- That there will be HIV positive people responding for MC, such people need counselling and ART to be accessible.
- Sex after MC, may need to wait longer than the 30 days followed in the studies

3.4.4 Effectiveness of MC from Systematic reviews

From the 35 cross-sectional studies in a Cochrane systematic review and meta-analysis of studies (Siegfried, *et al.,* 2007), the relative risk for HIV infection was 44% lower in circumcised men. Another meta-analytic review of studies from Sub- Sahara Africa (Weiss, *et al.,* 2000) noted a reduced risk of HIV infection in circumcised men of 0.42 (95% CI 0.34- 0.54%). The above reviews preceded the RCT's already discussed, whose results are consistent. On the basis of these findings, policy makers may rely on this evidence to propose interventions that reduce HIV infections in men.

3.4.5 MC from a wider social economic context

A lot has been written in observational studies conducted in Africa and Asia on MC. Evidence from cross-sectional studies demonstrates higher HIV prevalence among uncircumcised men (Lavrey, *et al.,* 1999; Diallo, *et al.,* 1992). Even culturally performed MC offers protection from HIV infection (Shaffer, *et al.,* 2007). But some studies, also note higher HIV infections due to sex with prostitutes, being unskilled and having a history of poor genital ulcers as major risk factors (Auvert, *et al*., 2001; Diallo, *et al.,* 1992).

Arguments, such as (Talbott, 2007), note that, HIV in Sub-Sahara Africa is accelerated by prostitution, poverty and unprotected sex, with an increased number of sexual partners. He notes that, higher numbers of prostitutes in Sub-Saharan Africa compared to Europe and Northern Africa is the problem. He argues that, HIV cannot be reduced by targeting "single encounter transmissions" for which MC is designed to reduce. Consequently, he observes, MC cannot bring down the epidemic rates where there are multiple infections from the infected prostitutes.

The above argument does not require policy makers to exclude MC from their programmes, but they should design programmes that target high risk groups. Studies have demonstrated that MC reduces HIV infections in high risk men who are exposed to prostitutes, and where alcohol, drugs, and sex with non- spousal partners are risk factors (Auvert, *et al*., 2001; Lavrey, *et al.,* 1999). However, there is generally conclusive evidence that being uncircumcised increases ones chances of getting STIs and HIV (Lavrey, *et al.,* 1999; Mahendale, *et al*., 1996; Tyndall, *et al*., 1996; Diallo, *et al*., 1992).

Research is also emerging (Oferall, *et al*., 2007; Oferall, *et al.,* 2006) to indicate that, poor genital hygiene (penile wetness) among men enhances HIV transmission, even in circumcised men. There is still insufficient evidence on genital hygiene and HIV transmission, but it is an important element that can still be considered in the IEC package for men.

The lessons which policy makers can draw from here is that, much as MC is needed for reducing infection in men; over reliance on it alone as an intervention, cannot provide an exhaustive solution for protection against HIV/AIDS. This calls for a combination prevention strategy (Sawires, *et al*., 2007). Such a package needs inclusion of most scientifically sound evidence-based strategies that are known to reduce HIV/AIDS.

3.4.6 Neonatal MC

Neonatal MC is acceptable for all Muslim children since it is a mandatory Islamic act of purification (Ali, 2006, Abdu'r Razzaq, 1998). There are more opportunities provided by neonatal MC compared to adult MC because it is cheaper and safer to conduct (Fergusson, *et al.*, 2006; Schoen, *et al.*, 2006). A Ugandan study also suggests a greater protective effect of MC at the pre-puberty stage (Kelly, *et al.,* 1999). In addition, neonatal MC is also worth considering because it protects the infants from other urinary tract infections as compared to uncircumcised infants (Fergusson, *et al.,* 1988; Wiswell, *et al.,* 1985). These findings should guide public health workers on when to offer MC and its long term benefits in reducing infection.

However, some of the neonatal studies above were conducted in the USA and New Zealand, with an advanced resource base that is not replicable in Africa. It would also be of interest to ascertain whether the mainly conservative Christian parents in some African settings like Uganda, would consent to neonatal MC for their children.

Table 9: Advantages and disadvantages of MC

Advantages	Disadvantages
Reduces HIV infection	Pain if without anaesthesia
Reduces STIs infection	Infections with poor care
Promotes penile hygiene	Irreversible operation
Therapeutic for phimosis and balanitis	Reduced sexual pleasure to some people

A one-off operation	May increase risk compensation
Neonatal MC possible	Not popular with all cultures
Healing 2- 4 weeks	Risks of excessive bleeding
Lower risk of penile cancer	Mainly male based intervention
Female Partners have lower risk of cancer of the cervix (WHO/UNAIDS,2007)	High Costs of implementation

Source: Author

3.4.7 Acceptability of MC in communities

MC is generally acceptable among different communities, despite the risks, if it is provided free (or at a substantially reduced cost), and in a hospital environment. In Botswana and Zimbabwe, MC was found to be acceptable among the young people, because of the associated health benefits (Halperin, *et al.,* 2005; Kababetstwe, *et al*., 2003). There have not been many acceptability studies on of MC in Uganda. But a section of Uganda's religious and cultural settings support it.

On the other hand, there are arguments against MC that it takes away the most sensitive parts of the male penis. They argue that, it ablates junctional mucosa which is an important component of the overall sensory mechanism of the human penis (Sorrell, *et al.*, 2006; Taylor & Taylor, 1996).

Some scholars also note that, MC robs the penis of its natural disposition for many motions of sexual pleasure (Kim & Pang, 2007). This also endangers the women, with hazards like abrasion, small raptures, tears in the vaginal wall and in some instances bleeding and severe pain (Gollaher, 1999). Such assertions are not very convincing, since they are not backed up by sufficient evidence. However, safeguards need to be in place to ensure that MC is safe for men and women.

It worth noting that, MC was found to be acceptable in men and women in Nyanza province of Kenya, who said that they would recommend it for their husbands and even male children (Baily, *et al.*, 2002).

3.4.8 Acceptability of MC among women

MC is also an opportunity for reducing HIV infection in women. But, much as it may reduce infection in men, women and children, over reliance on it may divert most resources to HIV prevention in men. This would leave fewer resources and attention to women focussed interventions. Women still have higher HIV prevalence and a greater vulnerability to STI infections than men (UNAIDS 2006). Women do not have an exclusively female controlled HIV prevention method. The female condom has not been popular with women in Uganda (The New Vision, 2007). There is also the fact that, women are highly vulnerable to HIV because their power to negotiate for safer sex with their male spouses is very limited (Mpagi, 2005). This is worsened by higher risks from infection, STIs and social degradation.

But in a study carried out in Kenya, women generally showed acceptance for MC. They noted that, MC was crucial in enhancing hygiene among men. In addition, CSWs noted that uncircumcised men always tear the condom and MC made it easier for men to wear condoms (Baily, *et al*., 2002).

3.4.9 International acceptance of MC

In response to the available evidence on MC, a joint WHO/UNAIDS communication has given its cautious approval. The response notes the following programme and policy implications (WHO/UNAIDS, 2007):

- MC should not replace the known methods for HIV prevention
- Countries should consider the need for IEC that is culturally sensitive
- Engage stakeholders on MC discussions
- Avail resources and proper costing for better MC
- MC should be gender sensitive by promoting gender equity, sexual health education for men and shared sexual decision making
- It should target high risk groups like adolescents and young men for maximum health benefit
- Identify countries' needs, training and consideration of local practices to improve safety
- Not recommended for HIV positive men

- Additional research is needed to inform the development of MC

The above pointers indicate a positive response from WHO and UNAIDS. However, the key issues addressed are developing country specific policies and programmes which need a lot of discussion and assessment. The statements above provide a good starting point for developing such policies and programmes. But some propositions on providing MC are not realistic, considering that the countries greatly affected are very poor.

USAID, in its published consensus of opinions from international researchers also recognises the benefits, programmatic and research implications of MC (USAID/AIDSMARK, 2002).

From the literature above, there is evidence that MC provides a degree of protection against HIV to circumcised men. If the opportunities identified are assessed and challenges addressed, MC can be a useful public health intervention. The opportunities provided by MC can also be integrated in the HIV/AIDS policy options already discussed.

This relationship between MC and HIV/AIDS is also summarised in figure 3 below which depicts the likely changes that may arise with the introduction of MC, within the framework of policies discussed. The issues considered take into consideration opportunities and challenges. A further discussion of the challenges thereafter seeks to see the problem in a broader outlook.

Figure 2: Prospective relationships between policies, practices and MC

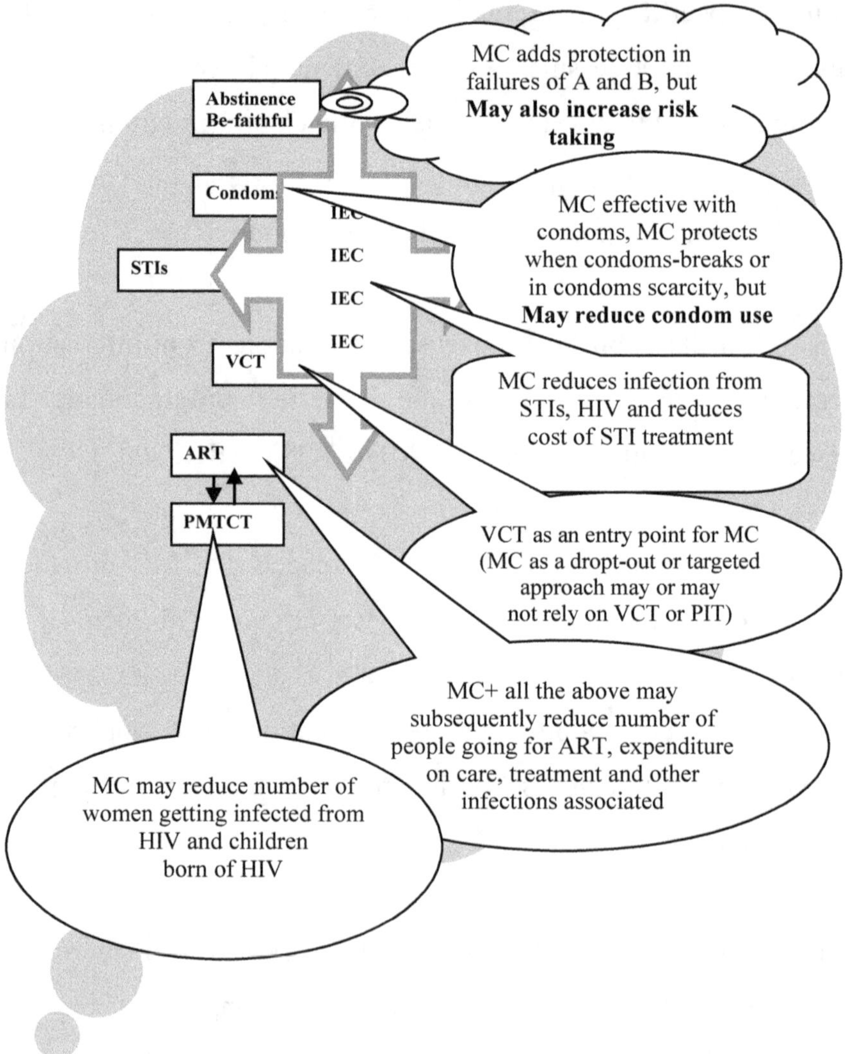

Source: Author

3.5 Challenges

3.5.1 The costs of providing MMC

The findings that MC reduces HIV infection in men have created demand for this operation (The BBC, 2007; Wise, 2006). This necessitates public health workers to evaluate the costs and even benefits of MMC in comparison to the existing forms of interventions. For instance, can MMC be provided to the poor, free of charge or at an affordable cost? Estimates have been made (Kahn, *et al.,* 2006) based on the South African study (by Auvert, *et al.*, 2006) to suggest that 1000 circumcisions would avert 308 (80%) of new infections in 20 years. In addition, modelled implications of MC discussed by Beyer and Wilson (2007) suggest that, by circumcising half of the men in Kenya and Botswana (one third of those likely to be infected); overall prevalence could be halved over three decades. If this is compared to the costs that would be spent on HIV/AIDS, funding for MMC programmes would need proof that this is a cheaper and effective option.

Depending on the available options for HIV/AIDS intervention with an MC dimension, alternatives of what is effectively beneficial may be considered. For instance, Holtgrave (2007) has identified a targeted testing and counselling of HIV positive persons as being more beneficial and cost effective than mass patient screening. This would be context specific since some countries' resources are highly constrained, like the case of

Uganda (See 1.4.5 & 1.4.6). There are huge costs that would be needed to train health and health care providers, and buy resources in order to provide a good service.

3.5.2 Consent, Ethical practice and human rights

Consent is defined as "agreeing, to give permission, to accede; to comply" and informed consent is based on "full information on what will happen" (Pearson Educational Limited, 2003). For the purpose of MC, it is important to consider issues of respect for autonomy, beneficence and justice. Autonomy gives the patient the right to make free decision; beneficence promotes the moral basis for practice by inflicting no harm, preventing harm, removing harm and promoting good; justice on the other hand, means that, people will be treated with fairness, appropriately and equitably (Mayberry and Mayberry, 2003). Consent may also be guided by ethical guidelines of medicine, such as the capacity to consent (age, maturity and cognitive ability), voluntariness and patients receiving sufficient information to guide consent (Macrae, 2007). There is always need to consider consent for vulnerable groups, defined as those (Macrae, 2007: 2) "without the capacity (relative, absolute or temporary) to give voluntary consent because of being disadvantaged educationally, economically or are physically impaired…"

The BMA guidelines highlight aspects of implementing neonatal MC. These include good practice, the law, consenting for children's best interests, uniform standards and human rights. They affirm human rights, which uphold basic principles like; not subjecting people to torture, rights to liberty and security, freedom of conscience and religion. These call for balancing conflicting rights and consulting with patients and their families. When implementing MC, considerations need to be taken into account on whether decisions impact on people's physical, economic, cultural, and other rights (The BMA, 2006). Such guidelines need to be context specific to work in Uganda.

On the other hand, when dealing with different groups' sexual health issues, for example adolescents, there may arise numerous challenges in decision making. An initiated communication between adolescents and their parents as they are provided with confidential care would resolve some issues (Summers, *et al.*, 2006). It should be recognised that, in the process of implementing MC, ethical issues will come up at neo-natal, preadolescent and post adolescent levels (Rennie, *et al.*, 2007).

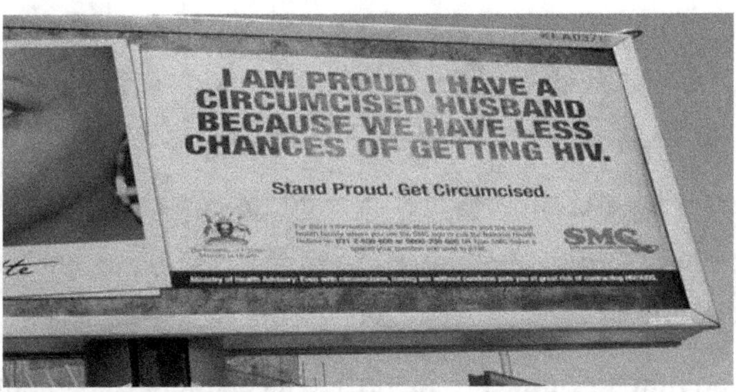

Plate 3: Campaign Communication post in Kampala, Uganda (Source Author)

Table 10: Opportunities and Challenges of providing MC

Level	Opportunities	Challenges
Community	• Political, cultural, religious, social acceptance of MC will promote its benefits to children, women and even men who do not get it. • Improving social structures- education, gender sensitive, ethical programmes based on human rights and policies sensitive to people's way of life.	• Poor resources in health institutions, poorly trained health workers; high health care costs may fail HIV/AIDS/MC related programmes. • Social opposition – from cultural, political and the religious
Individual	• Neo - natal, acceptability of MC at personal level reduces HIV Infection • MC process is a good moment for involving men in a "transformative SH education" like, "every man has a role as an individual to improve his lifestyle for the spouse's safety".	• High Individuals costs of MC if it is not subsidized or provided free. • Risk taking after MC is a personal issue that can increase HIV infection

Source: Author

3.6 Conclusion

In this chapter, I have discussed the evidence from three RCTs conducted in a clinical (medical) setting and two systematic reviews on the effectiveness of MC. I have also made an analysis of MC from a wider social context, looked at the neonatal and acceptability of MC (from women, communities and international organizations). All these are viewed as opportunities that can facilitate MC's implementation. On the other hand, the costs that may be involved vis-à-vis the health benefits and issues of consent, ethics and human rights are identified as challenges. A summarised analysis is made in table 10 above. In the next chapter, I propose policy options for appraisal, arising from my discussion of this and the previous chapters, based on set criteria.

4. CHAPTER FOUR

4.1. Introduction

In the foregoing chapter, I have discussed literature on MC with credible demonstration that, it provides a protective effect in men against HIV and STIs. That is the basis for making policy propositions below for future public health intervention. These propositions are appraised based on set criteria and some are highly recommended for their feasibility.

4.2. MMC and HIV/AIDS Policy options for consideration

Some of these options can be considered in case of implementing a comprehensive HIV/AIDS policy that is inclusive of MMC. In the description of these policy options, the following criteria are proposed as guideline (See table 12 for details).

Table 11: Criteria for policy appraisal and ranking

Criteria	Description/ranking
Technical feasibility	Expected outcome in terms of reducing infection

Financial feasibility	Willingness to fund from donors or government
Organizational feasibility	Ability to implement programme with other sectors
Social cultural feasibility	Acceptance from political, religious, women and cultural
Operational feasibility	Ease of implementation, budgeting, timing and monitoring
Feasibility rating	Highly feasible 3, very feasible 2, feasible 1, not feasible 0

Source: Author

4.3. Neonatal MC

This is of high technical feasibility and would give better protection (Kelly, *et al.*, 1999)). However, some medical personnel perceive neonatal MC as difficult to perform (Baily, *et al.*, 2002) as compared to adult MC. This would require training medical personnel to carry out operations in institutions.

Financially, this is the cheapest option of them all (Schoen, *et al.*, 2006). It can be funded by funding agencies and even from national budgets.

Organizationally, it can be provided as a drop-out service in public and private health facilities after birth. It can also be integrated into ANC education or the PMTC services offered to mothers. Private Health facilities (mainly Christian) may oppose it and consent from parents is crucial. But lessons can be drawn from the Muslim faith that has performed it for long.

For social – cultural and religious feasibility, it is highly accepted among the Uganda Muslims. Women have also shown its acceptance for the male children. In cultures where MC is an initiation rite to manhood, this may face some difficulties if it is offered at the neonatal stage

Operationally, it can be integrated into the institutional mechanisms of operation. This is feasible as part of the costs for ANC and PMTCT programmes already in place and can be monitored regularly.

4.4. MMC and ABC (14 - 24 years)

This is still technically feasible, as evident from table 7 and would provide continuity for those who would have missed MC at the earlier stages. This age bracket is a risk group which is vulnerable because of being sexually active.

Financially, the costs may be high for individuals seeking MMC and even condoms, if it is not subsidised, offered free by government or NGOs.

At organizational level, it can be organised with cultural institutions and NGOs. For school going children, MMC would be provided in the holidays and allow enough time for post operative care and healing. The FBOs, NGOs and politicians would continue with the ABC option.

For social – cultural and religious feasibility, it is acceptable since this is about the time boys attend initiation rites. Women still support it and at this level some people can give their own consent.

At operational level, it may be difficult to achieve continuity and proper schedules for operations. It is not easy to coordinate numbers of those willing to get MMC.

4.5. Targeted MC and Condoms (24 - 49 years)

Condoms and MMC provide a high Technical feasibility and would reduce the number of infection drastically. But among the sexually active group, it may encourage risk compensation which may compromise effectiveness.

Financially, this is feasible because the funding agencies would be willing to put money in a programme targeting a specific group for particular results. It would be expensive for individuals.

For social – cultural and religious feasibility, it is acceptable for the different social groups since it would seek their consent. Women also accept MC but have expressed fears that it would give men another excuse not to use condoms (Mail & Guardianonline, 2007)

In organization, the multi-sectoral approach to involve the district authorities, NGOs, and cultural institutions and societies is possible. Operationally, if organised as a programme, it would be very feasible and easier to monitor.

4.6. IEC with STI prevention and treatment messages

This is feasible, but some people do not respond to messages for behaviour change. But for the young people, specific messages have been known to work in Uganda where people have responded positively (Green, *et al.*, 2006).

Financially, this is fairly feasible because IEC has been in place, but needs better coordination of messages and sustained funding.

For social – cultural and religious, it is feasible and acceptable if IEC is packaged differently to benefit particular groups. IEC for MC among young people may be difficult without seeming to suggest that it does not give 100% protection.

In organization, multi-sectoral approach to involve the district authorities, NGOs, CBOs, the religious, cultural institutions and societies is possible. This can also highlight the options for prevention/treatment of STIs, VCT and ART and involving men in SH education.

At operational level, it is still hard to monitor performance. This may reduce further funding to the strategy.

4.7. VCT, MMC

Not highly technically feasible since fewer people have responded to the VCT services. VCT services may slow down MMC.

Financially, it is very expensive and the capacity to establish VCT services is not in place and may need greater commitment form donors. This is not feasible in the short term.

For social – cultural and religious feasibility, it has no opposition from the religious and cultures. It is feasible for women since it is part of ANC services in some countries.

With Organisation, it needs specialist training, structures in place to be implemented in the whole country. It is also difficult to implement, because it requires technical skills to manage.

Operationally, it is not very feasible because of uncertainty of people who may respond to the service in a given time but as routine ANC and PMTCT.

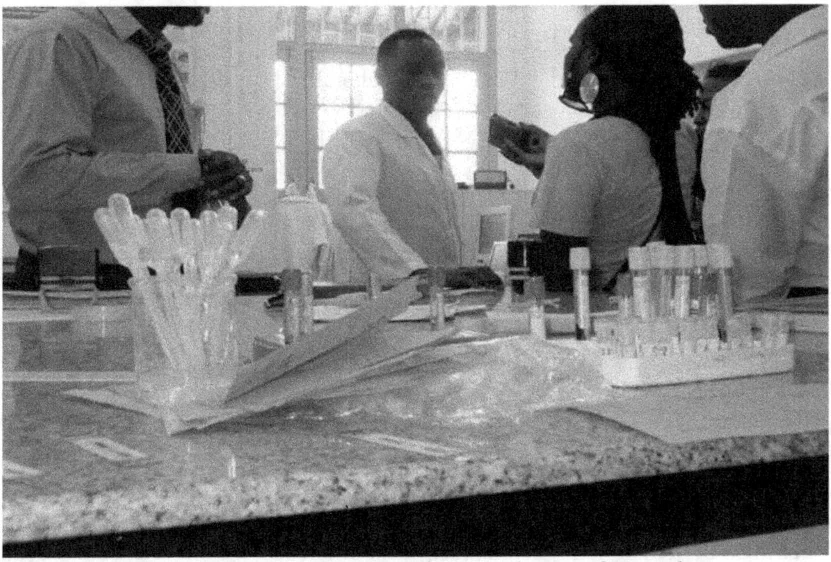

Plate 4: A mobile HIV-testing site set up in a rural area of Uganda (Source: Author)

4.8. MMC and HIV/AIDS Policy options for consideration

The above policy options description is summarised in the table below.

Table 12: Policy issues for consideration in MC implementation in HIV/AIDS

Strategic policy options	Technical feasibility	Financial Feasibility	Organizational Feasibility	Social - Cultural and religious	Operational Feasibility
(A). Neonatal MMC	Highly feasible; gives sustained protection	Highly feasible; can be financed from national budget	Highly feasible; As part of ANC/PMTCT for mothers	Very feasible; for Muslims and mothers, should address consent and cultural issues.	Highly feasible in hospitals, as part of institutional operations

(B). ABC & MMC (14-24)	Very feasible but needs delayed sex after MC, better post operative care and condom use	Feasible to fund from funding agencies with ABC	Very feasible with NGOs, cultural and other NGOs, Christian NGOs may oppose it	Feasible since MC is acceptable to Muslims, some cultures and women	Feasible but needs specific time planning for those in schools
(C).Targeted MMC and Condoms (25- 49)	Very feasible but needs delayed sex after MC, condoms and better care	Very feasible, Targeted MC can easily be funded.	Feasible, target group needs IEC for illiterates and conservative Christians	Feasible, adults can decide for themselves	Not feasible, uncoordinated Response for MC, unless proper schedules are in place
(D).IEC incorporating new MMC message, STI prevention and treatment	Feasible, though results may not be immediate	Feasible, but needs greater commitment	Feasible with collaboration of different stakeholders in design and promoting appropriate IEC	Feasible but needs to take into consideration other religious and cultural norms	Feasible but not very certain since it involves very many stakeholders, and indicators are obscure.
(E).MMC& VCT	Not feasible, uncertain if it can work, needs re-assessment	Simultaneous funding of these not feasible	Not feasible, VCT may slow down MC process	Feasible but some people may reject VCT as precondition for MMC	Feasible as component of ANC / PMTCT

Feasibility rating (See criteria in table 11)
Totals; A=14; B=7; C= 6; D=5; E= 2
Source: Author

4.9. Conclusion

In the above chapter, I have argued for the case of an opt-out neonatal MMC which should be given top priority. The other areas that need considerations are ABC & MMC (14-24), and targeted MMC supported with consistent condom use for (25 -49) for high risk populations. Evidently, other interventions that have been in place should continue, but some like VCT need to be reviewed. It is only the MMC element which needs a gradual integration into the whole process of HIV/AIDS prevention. This arises from the fact that it is new; there may be un-readiness to implement it and the need for a proper IEC within the different social cultural perception of Uganda. In the next chapter, I have made some recommendations directed at particular stake holders. I have also identified the context in which the new strategies are presumed to work for the communication plan suggested.

5. CHAPTER FIVE

5.1. Recommendations and conclusions

5.2 Introduction

In the previous chapter, I appraised the options available which call for a number of them to be taken up because HIV/AIDS needs different approaches to address it. But emphasis should be put on the ones that are more effective and give more certainty in bringing down the HIV prevalence over time. The recommendations suggested below are for adopting the effective options like neonatal MMC and MMC for different groups. But these are also in line with some approaches which have been in place like ABC, STI management and IEC. These are proposed to the stakeholders who are identified for key responsibilities.

5.3 Recommendations for key stakeholders

Table 13: Recommendations for integrating MC intervention to for stakeholders

Strategy	Recommendation	Responsibility	Time frame
Funding for MMC to make it affordable and accessible to	- Channel money to funding targeted MMC for persons of 14 – 24 & 25 -49 years - Ensure commitment to promoting IEC and condom	Donors and bilateral agencies	Medium term Medium term

those who need it	use - Propose better mechanism for monitoring HIV/AIDS funds		Medium term
Better IEC on HIV/AIDS, condoms and MMC through collaboration with other sectors	-Tone down attacks on condoms use and MC - Get informed about MMC - Involve all sectors in renewed HIV messages -Endorse MMC	Political and Local government leaders	Short term On – going On- going Short term
Assessment of capacity, Training staff and adopting MMC & IEC options	- Evaluate current operational capacity to carry out ethical neonatal M MC in institutions. -Provide health care staff with IEC on MMC - Identify resources that can provide MMC and on job training for surgeons to provide MMC in public institutions - Consider training cultural surgeons - Establish mechanism to monitor culturally performed MC - Integrate MC education in ANC - Offer neonatal MMC in all public institutions for consenting parents - Gradually adopt MMC for STIs/HIV prevention	Ministry of Health,	Medium term On-going Medium term Medium term Medium term Medium term Medium term Long term
Assessment, evaluation and research	- Analyse current VCT situation in a bid to improve it - Carry out further research on Culturally performed MC - Evaluate need for MMC among different age groups -Assess long term impact of MC on men - Continue research on effect of MC in HIV positive men on HIV negative women and MSM	Research bodies, health and health care bodies	Medium term Long term Long term Long term Long term

Recommendations (continued)

Strategy	Recommendation	Responsibility	Time frame
IEC – on MC and existing strategies; target high risk groups	- Target youths 14- 18 with renewed ABC and MC messages - Target women in urban and rural areas with specific SH messages eg. Encourage MMC -Incorporate penile hygiene, Condoms use messages for men and CSWs - Encourage men, women to attend STI clinics for treatment	NGOs and CBOs	Short term On - going Short term Short term
Better IEC – Adverts, radio talk shows, feature articles	- Report accurately about MC benefits i.e. not 100% effective - Report that MC works with condoms - Step up AB messages for young people 14- 18	The Media (FM radios, Television, English and vernacular newspapers)	Short term, short term short term
Improve upon the cultural practices	- Refer training for cultural surgeons to MOH - Call longer healing time after MMC (45 to 60 days) - Integrate behaviour change education in initiation customs before MC - Refer other MC to public institutions	Cultural institutions/Tribes	On going On going On going On going
Renew the AB campaigns	-Dialogue with partners on HIV/AIDS -Increase awareness on new scientific knowledge -Soften their stand on condom use	Religious leaders/ institutions	On going On going Short term

Source: Author

5.4 The context of policy implementation and challenges

The implementation suggested, involves a communication process that has simultaneous prevention strategies (Sawires, *et al.*, 2007). It is made on the assumption that the environment of the policy implementation comprises of different actors and processes that can achieve objectives by taking concern of broader society needs (Walt, 1994). This is simplified below:

Figure 3: The model for policy Implementation

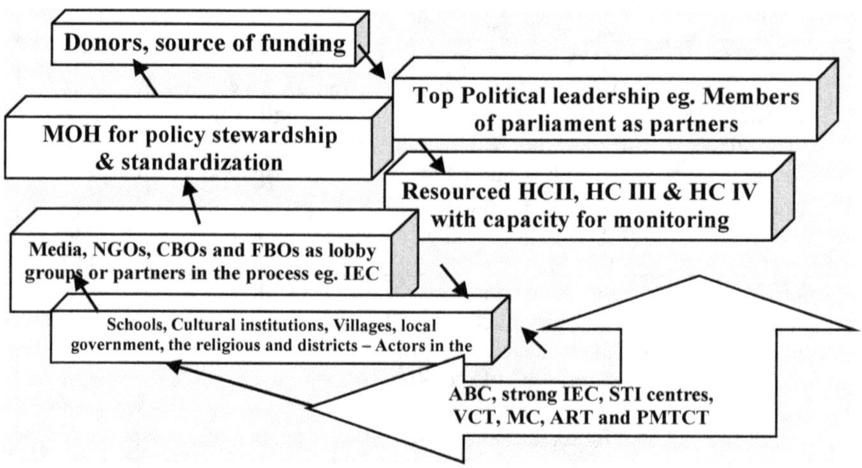

Source: Author, based on ideas by Walt (1994).

The structure, presented in figure 3 above, presumes that, the named sections in the context of the policy support each other to address the identified constraints below, for an effective delivery of needs related to HIV/AIDS. The options proposed need to be identifiable with the grassroots, recognising approaches like ABC, STI, VCT, ART, PMTCT and MC.

Table 14: Challenges expected and how to overcome them

Level	Expected challenge	How it can be addressed
1.Donors	Dictating their priorities	Agree on principles in SWAPS
2.Political leadership	Slow acceptance of MC	Adequately assess resistance/initiate dialogue
3.MOH	Lack of skills, insufficient resources	On job (peer) training, better costing
4.Research institutions	Lack of capacity to institute research	Seek collaboration with experts
5.NGOs, CBOs	Weak coordination	Workshops to demarcate roles
6.The media	Relaying wrong messages	Continuous involvement and correction
7.Cultural institutions	Refusal to refer other MC to hospitals	Train the local circumcisers well
8. The religious	May not endorse MC and condoms	Greater involvement, stick to A & B

Source: Author

5.5 The communication plan

This is a tentative communication plan which will be improved after consultations with partners involved at different policy levels in the country.

The communication process is based on the ESCR (2007) model. It involves making internal communications, media relations, public affairs, publicity materials and organising events. This includes checking perceptions, setting objectives, agreeing principles, developing messages and branding, prioritising audiences, choosing channels, estimating time, budget and evaluating success.

COMMUNICATION PLAN FOR HIV/AIDS – INCLUSIVE OF MC MESSAGE

Objective/ Content	Strategy/ activity	Target persons/ institutions	Activities	In-charge	Level place/ location	Likely challenges	Time frame	Monitoring indicator	Role of author
Support process of relaying a modified HIV/AIDS message with MMC	Internal communication	International partners, embassies, high commissions, Alliance Francais' and FORD Foundation	Report briefs delivery, budget proposals and description of activities	Embassy Secretaries of Alliance Francais and Ford contacts	Embassies and offices of associates named.	Availability of funds/ incorporating message in their programmes	2-3 months	Responses from the contacts identified	Improve communication plan, deliver plan as power point presentation
Evidence MMC in reducing HIV	Internal Communication and audience with key politician	The president, first lady, vice president and prime ministers	Letter writing to this power block, initiating dialogue	MOH, UNAIDS Uganda, ACP, TASO	Presidency, Ministerial level, top political level	Access to the politicians and their time limitations	1 – 3 months	Message delivery to the top politicians	Deliver findings to the in- charge by summarising sections of report

COMMUNICATION PLAN FOR HIV/AIDS – INCLUSIVE OF MC MESSAGE (Continued)

Objective/ Content	Strategy/ activity	Target persons/ institutions	Activities	In-charge	Level place/ location	Likely challenges	Time frame	Monitoring indicator	Role of author
Identify Opportunities of MC in the context of HIV/AIDS messages	Internal communication Report summary and recommendations	Health related professional bodies, CBOs, NGOS, TASO, ACP,MOH, AIC and other stakeholders	Relaying communication, discussion and analysis of briefs	Publicity secretaries of the named organizations and their contacts.	National (head offices), zonal organizations, district offices	Travel, identifying relevant organization that will be helpful	6 – 12 months	Groups that will be reached	Report writing, making short and clear messages from report
To appreciate Evidence of MC, advantages and disadvantages in context of HI V/AIDS	Summary of evidence and opportunities and challenges of MC	Members of parliament (Select committee on HIV/AIDS)	Summary of content, delivery of messages to select committee	Parliamentary press secretary and other staff	Parliament of Uganda, Kampala Uganda.	Members of parliament may not publicise this message, it being not political capital	4 - 8 months	Messages delivered to Members of parliament	Appointment with parliamentary press secretary to coordinate message delivery

COMMUNICATION PLAN FOR HIV/AIDS – INCLUSIVE OF MC MESSAGE (Continued)

Objective/ Content	Strategy/ activity	Target persons/ institution	Activities	In-charge	Level place/ location	Likely challenges	Time frame	Monitoring indicator	Role of author
Inform about ABC and MC, penile hygiene for men, VCT and ART	Media relations - Talk shows, brief adverts and songs	Media – TV, FM radio, English and vernacular newspapers	TV and radio talk shows, developing messages	Partners like ACP, NGOs involved in HIV/AIDS	Media houses nationwide	Expenses on media waves may be expensive	On-going	Number of messages aired and talks hosted. Feeds back through call in	Write a feature article in the Monitor Newspape
Know opportunitie s and challenges of MC in context of HIV/AIDS	Written summary of report and recommenda tions	The district authorities, local government representativ es	Distribution of report and meeting with key persons at the district	Associates like NGOs and those involved in HIV/AIDS	Districts, regions, local government	Costs, access to districts and failure of districts to support process	4- 6 months	Messages delivered to districts and responses of districts	Deliver message to local government committees on health

COMMUNICATION PLAN FOR HIV/AIDS – INCLUSIVE OF MC MESSAGE (Continued)

Objective/ Content	Strategy/ activity	Target persons/	Activities	In-charge	Level place/ location	Likely challenges	Time frame	Monitoring indicator	Role of author
Know about MC as an added advantage in prevention of STIs and HIV/AIDS / need for neonatal MC.	Publicity materials- Pamphlets, leaflets and posters with benefits of MC	Health and health care professionals in government and NGOs or FBOs	Design of messages, discussion and distribution	Partners like MOH	Health and Health care facilities	Slowness of MOH to effect communication	4 – 8 months	Number of messages given to health and healthcare workers	Write brief for MOH policy department
Know opportunities and challenges of MC, the need for neonatal MC in ABC, VCT and STIs prevention	Communication and events with cultural institutions	Heads of cultural institutions, cultural and tribes that practice MC (traditional surgeons)	Letters, meetings, seminars and cultural dinners	Representatives from the HIV/AIDS partners	Community level	Acceptance from cultural institutions and surgeons	2- 6 months	Number of cultural institutions visited	observer in message formulation process for cultural institutions

NB: An additional communication plan to the one above, will target tertiary Institutions, like universities (18 – 49 years), secondary schools (14 – 18 years, Rural and urban women groups; urban uneducated men living in slums and CSWs; religious leaders and urban working educated men. Each of these groups will have a specific message, which is suited to their culture and environment.

5.4 Conclusion

In conclusion, this study has provided me with the opportunity to assess intervention approaches of reducing HIV infections from a new dimension. My fear is that, it is an intervention riddled with so many controversies. The most challenging part of the MC policy is its implementation without behaviour dis-inhibition. That is why the success of the programme, (14 – 49 years), will highly depend on an effective communication that encourages correct and consistent use of condoms.

The hope for MC also stems from the support of WHO, UNAIDS, BINGO's and Multilateral agencies like USAID. As for the BONGO's, it perhaps robs them of profits that would be made from condom sales. For governments like that of Uganda, it is a new surgical intervention that may have an enormous implication on the health of others (including women, children). But if options like neonatal and adult MC are provided because of their benefits, can the capacity (human, financial) be created to sustain the programme? It is also important to bring aboard the religious, women, men and cultural institutions.

Fortunately, evidence suggests that MC is effective in reducing infections from STIs and HIV. And countries of Sub-Saharan Africa, ravaged by deaths from HIV/AIDS may not afford to be occupied in arguments of reduced sexual pleasure due to MC. HIV/AIDS is also still a complex issue that does not need just one approach to address it. Reducing HIV/AIDS infections needs everything else that works.

With scientific knowledge at hand, is it becomes unethical to deny people, an intervention which is almost as effective as a vaccine. Perhaps, if MC had been adopted 20 years ago, the epidemic would have been halved by now. Unfortunately, there are still a lot of bureaucratic hurdles to overcome.

REFERENCES

Abdu'r Razzaq, A.B. (1998) Circumcision in Islam. London: Dar Al Taqua Ltd.

Ali, K. (2006) Sexual ethics and Islam: Feminist reflections on Qu'ran. Hadith and Jurisprudence. Oxford: One World publications.

Auvert, B.,Buve,A., Lagarde,E.,Kahindo,M.,Chege,J.,Rutenberg,N.,*et al.* (2001), Male Circumcision and HIV infection in four cities in Sub- Saharan Africa. *AIDS* [Online] 15(suppl.4), S31-S40. Available from World Wide Web: <http://www.aidsonline.com/pt/re/aids/> [28 May 2007].

Auvert,B.,Taljaard,D.,Lagarde,E.,Sobngwi-Tambekou,J.L.,Sitta.R.,*et al.* (2005) Randomized Controlled Intervention Trial of Male Circumcision for Reduction of HIV Infection Risk: The ANRS 1265 Trial. *Plos medicine* [Online] 2(11), e298. 1112-1122. Available from World Wide Web: <http://medicine.plosjournals.org/archive/15491676/2/11/pdf/10.1371_journal.pmed.0020298-L.pdf> [26 February 2007].

Bailey,R.C.,Moses,S.,Parker,B.C.,Agot,K.,Maclean,I.,Krieger,J.N., *et al.* (2006) Male Circumcision for HIV prevention in young men in Kisumu, Kenya: a randomised controlled trial. *The Lancet* [Online] 369 (9562), 643- 656. Available from World Wide Web: <http://0-www.sciencedirect.com.wam.leeds.ac.uk/ > [26 February 2007].

Baily.R.C., Muga,R.,Poulussen,R.,Abicht,H. (2002) The acceptability of male circumcision to reduce HIV infections in Nyanza province, Kenya. [Online] *Aids Care* 14 (1), 27-40. Available from World Wide Web: <http://www.informaworld.com/ > [20 June 2007].

Bass, E. (2005) Fighting to close the condom gap in Uganda. *The Lancet* [Online] 365(9465),1127-1128. Available from World Wide Web: <http://0-www.sciencedirect.com.wam.leeds.ac.uk/> [29 May 2007].

Belated, but powerful: The response of the catholic church to HIV/AIDS in five Southern African Countries. (2007) [Online] CAFOD. Available from the World Wide Web: <http://www.cafod.org.uk/var/storage/original/application/phpOwS4s4.pdf> [Accessed 20 May 2007].

Beyer,J & Wilson,D. (2006) Male circumcision: Evidence and implications, HVI/AIDS M&E, getting the results series, [Online] Reports produced for the World Bank Global HIV/AIDS programme. Available from the World Wide Web: <http://siteresources.worldbank.org/INTHIVAIDS/Resources/375798-1132695455908/M&EGR_MaleCircumcision_Mar31.pdf/> [Accessed 9 July 2007].

Buvé, A. (2002) HIV Epidemics in Africa: What Explains the Variations in HIV Prevalence? *IUBMB Life*[Online] 53(4), 193 – 195. Available from World Wide Web: <http://dx.doi.org/10.1080/15216540212641/> [21 May 2007].

Circumcision: A woman's view. (2007)[Online]. Mail & Guardianonline. Available from the World Wide Web: <http://www.mg.co.za/articlePage.aspx?articleid=311625&area=/insight/monitor> [Accessed 20 June, 2007].

Collins, T (2005) "Health Policy analysis: A simple tool for policy makers. *Public Health* [Online] 119(3), 192- 196. Available from World Wide Web

:<http://www.sciencedirect.com.wam.leeds.ac.uk/> [3 August 2007].

Core Health Indicators; Country information. (2005a) [Online]. WHO. Available from the World Wide Web: <http://www.who.int/whosis/database/core/core_select_process.cfm> [Accessed 22.May 2007].
Demographic and socio-economic data. Uganda HIV indicators (2005) [Online]. WHO. Available from the World Wide Web: <http://www.who.int/hiv/HIVCP_UGA.pdf> [Accessed 6th April 2007].

Diallo, O.M.,Ackah,N.A.,Lafontaine,M.F.,Doorly.D.,Roux.R.,Kanga.J.M., *et al*. (1992) HIV-1 and HIV-2 infections in men attending sexually transmitted disease clinics in abidjan, Cote d'Ivoire. *AIDS.* 6(6), 581-585.

Drain, K.P., Smith,J.S, Hughes,J.P., Halperin,D.T and Holmes,K.K. (2004) Correlates of National HIV Seroprevalence: An Ecological Analysis of 122 Developing Countries. [Online] *J Acquir Immune Defic Syndr.* 35(4), 407–420. Available from World Wide Web: <http://www.medscape.com/viewpublication/> [21 May 2007].

Eaton, L. (2005) Global Fund pulls funds to Uganda and Myanmar. [Online] *British Medical Journal*. [Online] 331(7515), 475. Available from World Wide Web: <http://0-www.bmj.com.wam.leeds.ac.uk/> [6 July 2007].

Eaton, L. (2005a) Global Fund toughens stance against corruption. *British Medical Journal*. [Online] 331(7519), 718. Available from World Wide Web: <http://0-www.bmj.com.wam.leeds.ac.uk/> [6 July 2007].

Fergusson,D.M.,Boden,J.M. & Horwood, J.L. (2006) Circumcision status and risk of sexually transmitted infections in young adult males: An analysis of a longitudinal birth cohort. *Pediatrics*

[Online] 118(5), 1971-1975. Available from World Wide Web: <http://pediatrics.aappublications.org/cgi/reprint/118/5/1971> [6 July 2007].

Fergusson,M.,Lawton,J.M.,Shannon,F.T. (1988) Neonatal Circumcision and Penile Problems: An 8-Year Longitudinal Study. *Paediatrics* [Online] 81(4), 537-541D. Available from World Wide Web: <http://pediatrics.aappublications.org/cgi/reprint/81/4/537> [6 July 2007].

Frammer, M and Rychetnik L. (2003) From Evidence based medicine to evidence based public health. In: V.Lin and B. Gibson (eds.) Evidence based Health Policy. New York: Oxford University Press. pp.56-69.

Gollaher,D.L (1999) Circumcision: A history of the world's most controversial surgery. New York: Basic books.

Gray, R. H G., Kigozi, G., Serwadda,D., Makumbi, F.R.,Watya, S. *et al.* (2006) Male Circumcision for HIV prevention in men in Rakai, Uganda: a randomised trial. *The Lancet* [Online] *369* (9562), 657- 666. Available from World Wide Web: <http://0-www.sciencedirect.com.wam.leeds.ac.uk:80/> [12 March 2007].

Green,E.C.,Halperin,D.,Nantulya,V.,Hogle,J.A. (2006) Uganda's HIV prevention success: The role of sexual behaviour change and the national response. *AIDS and Behaviour*. [Online] 10 (4), 335-346. Available from World Wide Web: <http://www.pubmedcentral.nih.gov/picrender.fcgi?artid=1544373&blobtype=pdf> [28 May 2007].

Halperin, D.T., Fritz, K., McFarland, W., Woelk, G. (2005) Acceptability of Adult Male Circumcision for Sexually Transmitted Disease and HIV Prevention in Zimbabwe. *Sex Transm Dis* [Online] 32(4), 238-9. Available from World Wide Web: <http://gateway.uk.ovid.com. wam.leeds.ac.uk /> [16 July 2007].

Holtgrave,D.R. (2007) Costs and Consequences of the US Centers for Disease Control and Prevention's Recommendations for Opt-Out HIV Testing. *PloS Medicine* [Online] 4(6), 1011 – 1018. Available from World Wide Web: <http://medicine.plosjournals.org/archive/1549-1676/4/6/pdf/10.1371_journal.pmed.0040194-L.pdf> [18 July 2007].

Human Rights Watch Reacts To Uganda Aids, Uganda should be building on its success, not adopting the United States' failures. (2005) [Online] Human Rights Watch. Available from the World Wide Web: <http://hrw.org/reports/2005/uganda0305/1.htm> [Accessed 23rd May, 2007].

Jacobs, B., Kambugu, F. S. K., Whitworth, J. A.G., Ochwo. M., Pool. A. R., Lwanga. A., *et al.* (2003) Social marketing of pre-packaged treatment for men with urethral discharge (*Clear Seven*) in Uganda. *International Journal of STD & AIDS* [Online] 14(3), 216–221. Available from World Wide Web: <http://0-docserver.ingentaconnect.com.wam.leeds.ac.uk/> [4 June 2007].

Jeppsson, A. (2001) Financial priorities under decentralization in Uganda. *Health Policy and planning.* [Online] 16 (2), 187-192.Availavle from World Wide Web : <http://heapol.oxfordjournals.org/cgi/reprint/16/2/187> [25 April 2007].

Kahn,J.G.,Marseille,E., Auvert, B. (2006) Cost-Effectiveness of Male Circumcision for HIV Prevention in a South African Setting. *PlosMedicine* [Online]. 3(12), e517. 2349-2358. Available from World Wide Web: <http://medicine.plosjournals.org/perlserv/?request=getdocument&doi=10.1371/journal.pmed.0030517> [10 March 2007].

Kebaabetswe, P., Lockman, S., Mogwe, S., Mandevu, R., Thior, I., Essex, M., *et al*, (2003) Male circumcision: an acceptable strategy for HIV prevention in Botswana. *Sex Transm Infect* [Online]

79(3),214–219. Available from World Wide Web: <http://sti.bmj.com/cgi/reprint/79/3/214> [28 May 2007].

Kelly,R..,Kiwanuka,N.,Wawer,M.J.,Serwadda,D.,Sewankambo,N. K.,Mangheni,W.F.,Li, C., *et al*. (1999) Age of male circumcision and risk of prevalent HIV Infection in rural Uganda. *AIDS* [Online]13(3), 399-405. Available from World Wide Web: <http://gateway.uk.ovid.com/gw1/ovidweb.cgi?/> [26 June 2007].

Kim,D & Pang,M.G. (2007). The effect of male circumcision on sexuality. *BJU international* [Online] 99(3), 619 – 622]. Available from World Wide Web: <.http://0-www.blackwell-synergy.com.wam.leeds.ac.uk/> [16 July 2007].

Krieger,J.N.,Baily,C.R.,Opeya,J.,Ayieko,B.,Opiyo,F.,Kawango,A., *et al.* (2005) Adult male circumcision: Results of a standardized procedure in Kisumu District, Kenya. *BJU International* [Online] 96(7), 1109-1113. Available from the Wide World Web: <http://0-www.blackwell-synergy.com.wam.leeds.ac.uk/> [28 May 2007].

Lavrey,L.,Rakwar,P.J.,Thompson,L.M.,Jackson,D.J.,Mandaliya,K. ,Chohan,H.B., *et al.* (1999), Effect of circumcision on incidence of Human Immunodeficiency virus type 1 and other sexually transmitted diseases: A prospective cohort study of trucking company employees in Kenya. *The Journal of Infectious Diseases* [online] 180(2),330-336. Available from World Wide Web: <http://www.journals.uchicago.edu/JID/journal/issues/v180n2/981351/981351.web.pdf> [29 May 2007].

Macrae,D.J. (2007) The Council for International Organizations and Medical Sciences (CIOMS) Guidelines on Ethics of Clinical Trials. *Proc Am Thorac Soc*[Online] 4(2),176-178.Available from World Wide Web: <http://pats.atsjournals.org/cgi/reprint/4/2/176> [3 June 2007].

Magoni, M., Okong, P., Bassani, L., Namaganda,K.P, Onyango, S., Giuliano, M. (2007) Implementation of a programme for the prevention of mother to child transmission of HIV in a Ugandan hospital over five years: challenges, improvements and lessons learned. *Int J STD AIDS.* [Online] 18(2), 109-13. Available from World Wide Web: <http://0-www.ingentaconnect.com.wam.leeds.ac.uk/> [22 May 2007].

Maharaj,P. (2006) Reasons for Condom Use Among Young People In KwaZulu-Natal: Prevention of HIV, Pregnancy or Both? *International Family Planning Perspectives* [Online] 32(1),28–34. Available from World Wide Web: <http://www.guttmacher.org/pubs/journals/3202806.html> [22 May 2007].

Mahendale,S.M.,Shepherd.E.M.,Divekar,A.D.,Gangakhedkar.R.R., Kamble, S.Smenon, P.A, *et al.* (1996) Evidence for high prevalence and rapid transmission of HIV among individuals attending STD clinics in Pune, India. *Indian J of medical Res*, 104, 327-335.

Manuel, S. (2005) Obstacles to condom use among secondary school students in Maputo city, Mozambique.*Cult Health Sex* [Online] 7(3), 293 – 302. Available from World Wide Web: <http://0-www.informaworld.com.wam.leeds.ac.uk/> [7 June 2007].

Matovu,K.B.,Gray,R.H.,Makumbia,F.,Wawerc,J.M.,Serwadda,D., Kigozi,G, *et al.* (2005) Voluntary HIV counselling and testing acceptance, sexual risk behavior and HIV incidence in Rakai, Uganda. *AIDS* [Online] 19 (5), 503–511.Available from World Wide Web: <http://0-gateway.uk.ovid.com.wam.leeds.ac.uk/> [15 June 2007].

Matovu,K.B.J.,Kigozi,G.,Nalugoda,F.,Wabwiremangheni,F.,Gray, H.R. (2002) The Rakai Project counselling programme experience. [Online] 7(12), 1064–1067.Available from World Wide Web: <http://0-gateway.uk.ovid.com.wam.leeds.ac.uk/> [December 2002].

Mayberry, M and Mayberry,J. (2003) Consent in clinical practice. Abingdon: Radcliffe Medical press.

McConnel, C.E., Stanley, N., Du Plessis, J.A., Pitter., C.S., Abdulla, F., Coovadia., H.M., Marseille, E., Kahn, J.G.(2005) The cost of a rapid-test VCT clinic in South Africa.*South Africa Medical Journal* [Online] 95(12), 968-971.Available from World wide web: <http://blues.sabinet.co.za/WebZ/Authorize?/> [2 June 2007].

Mitchell,K., Nakamanya,S.,Kamali,A.,Whitworth,J.A. (2001) Community based HIVAIDS education in rural Uganda, Which channel is most effective? *Health Education research.* [Online] 16(4), 411–423. Available from World Wide Web: < http://her.oxfordjournals.org/cgi/reprint/16/4/411> [22 May 2007].

Mpagi,S.J (2005) Is ABC message still effective in the contemporary Uganda? A social- cultural and gender perpective, In: The 3rd session of the Uganda Think tank on AIDS (UTTA), Grand Imperial Hotel, Kampala, 14th July, 2005.UTTA.

Muhwava,W. (2004) Condom Use within Marriage and Consensual Unions in the Era of HIV/AIDS in Zimbabwe. *African Population Studies* [Online] 19(1), 119-14. Available from World Wide Web: <http://www.bioline.org.br/request?ep04007> [28 May 2007].

Mukenge-Tshibaka, L., Alary, M., Geraldo, N., Lowndes, C.M.(2005) Incorrect condom use and frequent breakage among female sex workers and their clients. *International Journal of STD & AIDS* [Online] 16 (5), 345 -347. Available from World Wide Web: <http://0-www.ingentaconnect.com.wam.leeds.ac.uk/> [30 May, 2007].

Namutebi,J. (2007) Government attacked over expired female condoms [Online] The New Vision. Available from the World Wide Web:< http://www.newvision.co.ug/D/8/13/569707> [Accessed 10 June 2007].

Ofarrell.N. (1999) Increasing prevalence of genital herpes in developing countries:implications for heterosexual HIV transmission and STI control programmes. *Sexually Transmitted Infections [*Online] 75(6), 377-84. Available from World Wide Web: <http://0-sti.bmj.com.wam.leeds.ac.uk/> [1 June 2007].

Oferall,N.,Morison,L and Chung,C. (2007) Low Prevalence of Penile Wetness Among Male Sexually Transmitted Infection Clinic Attendees in London. *Sexually Transmitted* Diseases. [Online] 34(6),408–409. Available from World Wide Web: <http://0-gateway.uk.ovid.com.wam.leeds.ac.uk/> [28 June 2007] .

Oferall, N.,Morison,L.,Moodley,P.,Pillay,K.,Vanmali,T.,Quigley,M.,Hayes ,R and Sturm,.A. W. (2006) Association Between HIV and Subpreputial Penile Wetness in Uncircumcised Men in South Africa .*Journal of Acquired defic syndrome* [Online] 43(1), 69-77. Available from World Wide Web: <http://0-gateway.uk.ovid.com.wam.leeds.ac.uk/> [28 June 2007].

Okonkwo, K.C., Reich. K., Alabi, A.I., Umeike, N., Nachman, S.A.(2007) An evaluation of awareness: attitudes and beliefs of pregnant Nigerian women toward voluntary counseling and testing for HIV. *AIDS Patient Care STDS.* [Online] 21(4), 252-60. Available from World Wide Web: < http://www.liebertonline.com/doi/abs/10.1089/apc.2006.0065/> [22 may 2007].

Okware, S, (2005) Evidence based support for the ABC strategy. In: The 3rd session of the Uganda Think tank on AIDS (UTTA), Grand Imperial Hotel, Kampala, 14th July, 2005.UTTA.

Okware, S.,Kinsman.J.,Onyango.S.,Opio.A and Kaggwa.P. (2005) Revisiting the ABC strategy: HIV prevention in Uganda in the era of antiretroviral therapy. *Postgrad. Med.J* [online] 81 (960), 625-628. Available from World Wide Web: <http://0-pmj.bmj.com.wam.leeds.ac.uk/ > [11 May 2007].

Oyedirani,K.A. (2003) Determinants of condom use among monogamous men in Ondo State, Nigeria. *Journal of Health, Population and Nutrition* [Online] 21(4), 358-366. Available from World Wide Web: <http://www.icddrb.org/images/jhpn2104_determinants.pdf> [16 June 2007].

Parsons, D.W. (1995) Public policy: An Introduction to the theory and practice of policy analysis. Aldershot: Edward Elgar Publishing Limited.

Pearson Educational Limited, (2003) Longman dictionary of contemporary English, Essex: Longman.

Rennie, S.,Muula.S.A. and Westreich,D. (2007) Male circumcision and HIV prevention: ethical medical and public health tradeoffs in low-income countries. *J. Med. Ethics* [Online] 33(6), 357-361. Available from World Wide Web: <http://jme.bmj.com/cgi/reprint/33/6/357> [6 July 2007].

Report on the global AIDS epidemic; A UNAIDS. 10th anniversary special edition. (2006) [Online]. UNAIDS. Available from the World Wide Web: <http://data.unaids.org/pub/GlobalReport/2006/2006_GR-ExecutiveSummary_en.pdf> [Accessed 3rd July 2007].

Reynolds, S J., Risbud, A R., Shepherd, M E., Rompalo, A M ., Ghate, M V., Godbole, S V., Joshi, S N., *et al.* (2006) High rates of syphilis among STI patients are contributing to the spread of HIV-1 in India. *Sex. Transm. Inf.* 82(2),121-126. Available from World Wide Web: <http://0-sti.bmj.com.wam.leeds.ac.uk/> [6 July 2007].

Reynolds,J.S., Shepherd,M.E.,Risbud,A.R., Gangakhedkar,R.R.,Brookmeyer,R.S.,Divekar, A.D., Mehendale,M.S., Bollinger.RC. (2004) Male circumcision and risk of HIV-1 and other sexually transmitted infections in India. *The Lancet*[Online] 363 (9414), 1039–40. Available from World Wide

Web: <http://0-www.sciencedirect.com.wam.leeds.ac.uk/> [29 May 2007].

Rietmeijer, C.A.M., Krebs, J.W.,Feorino, P.M., and Judson, F.N. (1988) Condoms as physical and chemical barriers against Human Immunodeficiency Virus. *Journal of the American Medical Association.* 259 (12), 1851-1853.

Sadgrove, J. (2007) 'Keeping up appearances' Sex and religion amongst university students in Uganda. *Journal of religion in Africa.*[Online] 37(17), 116-144. Available from World Wide Web: <http://0-www.ingentaconnect.com.wam.leeds.ac.uk/> [28 May 2007].

Sawires,R.S., Dworkin, S.L., Fiamma,A., Peacock,D., Szekeres,G and Coates,T.J. (2007) Male Circumcision and HIV/AIDS: Challenges and opportunities. *The Lancet* [Online] 369 (9562), 708- 713. Available from World Wide Web: <http://0-www.sciencedirect.com.wam.leeds.ac.uk/> [5 March 2007].

Schoen, E.J., Colby, C.J & To, T.T. (2006) Cost analysis of neonatal circumcision in a large health maintenance organization. *J of Urol* [Online] 175(3), 1111-1115. Available from World Wide Web: <http://www.sciencedirect.com.wam.leeds.ac.uk/> [22 June 2007].

Serwadda, D., Gray,R.H.,Sewankambo,N.K., Wabwire-Mangen,F., Chen,M.Z.,. Quinn,T.C Lutalo,T., Kiwanuka,N., *et al.* (2003) Human Immunodeficiency Virus Acquisition Associated with Genital Ulcer Disease and Herpes Simplex Virus Type 2 Infection: A Nested Case-Control Study in Rakai, Uganda. *The Journal of Infectious Diseases* [online] 188(10),1492–7. Available from World Wide Web: <http://www.journals.uchicago.edu/JID/journal/issues/v188n10/30634/30634.web.pdf> [23 May 2007].

Shaffer,D.N.,.Bautista,T.C.,Sateren.,W.B.,Sawe,F.K.,Kiplangat,S. C.,Miruka,A.O.,Renzullo,O.P., *et al.* (2007)The protective effect of circumcision on HIV incidence in rural low-risk men circumcised predominantly by traditional circumcisers in Kenya. *J Acquir Immune Defic Syndr* [Online] 45(4), 371–379. Available from World Wide Web: <http://gateway.uk.ovid.com/gw1/ovidweb.cgi?/> [31 August 2007].

Shuey,D.A.,Babishangire,B.B.,Omiat,S and Bagarukayo, H. (1999) Increased sexual abstinence among in-school adolescents as a result of Health Education in Soroti district, Uganda. *Health Education Research* [Online] 14 (3), 411-19. Available from World Wide Web: <http://her.oxfordjournals.org/cgi/reprint/14/3/411> [28 May, 2007].

Siegfried,N.,Muller, M.,Volmink.J. (2007) Male circumcision for prevention of heterosexual acquisition of HIV in men. *Cochrane Database of Systematic Reviews* [Online] 3. CD003362. DOI: 10.1002/14651858.CD003362. Available from World Wide Web: <http://www.mrw.interscience.wiley.com/cochrane/clsysrev/articles/CD003362/frame.html> [14 March 2007].

Singh, S. (2003) ABC, the roles of Abstinence, monogamy and Condom use. *Reproductive Health Matters* [Online] 12 (23), 129-131. Available from World Wide Web: <http://0-www.sciencedirect.com.wam.leeds.ac.uk/> [2 May 2007].

Sorrell, M.L., Snyder, J.L.,Reiss,M.D.,Eden,C.,Milos,F.M.,Wilcox,N and Howe.V.S.R. (2006) Fine touch pressure threshold in the adult penis. *BJU International*[Online] 99(4), 864-869. Available from World Wide Web: <http://0-www.blackwell-synergy.com.wam.leeds.ac.uk/> [29 July 2007].

Source disbursement. (2007) [Online]. The Global Fund. Available from the World Wide Web:<http://www.theglobalfund.org/Programs/Portfolio.aspx?countryID=UGD&lang=en> [Accessed 27 June 2007].

Stoneburner,R.L and Low-Beer, D. (2004) Avoidance in Uganda Population-Level HIV Declines and Behavioral Risk. *Science* [Online] 304(5671), 714-718. Available from World Wide Web: <http://www.sciencemag.org/cgi/reprint/304/5671/714.pdf> [8 June 2007].

Summers, D., Alpert, I., Rousseau-Pierre, T., Minguez, M., Manigault, S., Edwards, S., Nucci, A., Diaz, A. (2006) An Exploration of the Ethical,Legal and Developmental Issues in the Care of an Adolescent Patient. *Mt. Sinai Journal of Med* [Online] 73(3), 592-595. Available from World Wide Web: <http://www.mssm.edu/msjournal/73/73_3_pages_592_595.pdf> [4 July 2007].

Sweat, M., Gregorich, S., Sangiwa, G., Furlonge, C., Balmer, D., Kamenga, C., Grinstead, O., Coates, T. (2000) Cost effectiveness of VCT HIV counselling and testing in Kenya and Tanzania. *The Lancet* [Online] 356 (9224), 113-21. Available from World Wide Web: <http://0-www.sciencedirect.com.wam.leeds.ac.uk/> [16 June 2007].

Talbot,J.R.(2007) Size matters: The number of prostitutes and the global HIV/AIDS pandemic. [Online] *PLoS ONE* 2(6), e543. doi:10.1371/ journal.pone.0000543. Available from World Wide Web: <http://www.plosone.org/article/fetchArticle.action?articleURI=info:doi/10.1371/journal.pone.0000543> [28 June 2007].

Taylor,J.R., Lockwood, A.P., Taylor, A. J. (1996) The prepuce: specialized mucosa of the penis and its loss to Circumcision; *British Journal of Urology* [Online] 77(2), 291–295.Available from World Wide Web: < http://0-www.blackwell-synergy.com.wam.leeds.ac.uk/> [22 June 2007].

The law and Ethics of male circumcision – Guidance for doctors. (2006) [Online].BMA. Available from the World Wide Web: <http://www.bma.org.uk/ap.nsf/content/malecircumcision2006> [accessed 26 June 2007].

The Republic of Uganda (2001) Uganda Demographic and Health survey. Uganda bureau of statistics. Entebbe. Available from the World Wide Web <http://www.measuredhs.com/pubs/pdf/FR128/FR128.pdf> [Accessed 12 March 2007].

The Republic of Uganda. (1999) Uganda National Health policy. Kampala: Ministry of Health.

The Republic of Uganda. (2003) National Policy on Public Private partnership in Health, Final Editorial draft, Kampala: Ministry of Health.

The Republic of Uganda. (2003a) STD/HIV/AIDS Surveillance Report. Kampala: Ministry of Health,

The Republic of Uganda. (2004) National condom guidelines and strategy. Kampala: Ministry of Health.

The Republic of Uganda. (2006) The Uganda HIV/AIDS sero-behaviour survey 2004-2005. Kampala: Ministry of Health.

The Republic of Uganda, (2006a) Assessment manual for Higher and lower local government, Kampala: Ministry of Local government.

The Republic of Uganda, (2006b) Human resources for health policy. Kampala: Ministry of Health.

The Republic of Uganda (2007a) Ministry of Health, Health Infrastructure, Available on the World wide Web: <http://www.health.go.ug/health_units.htm> [Accessed 05 March 2007].

The New Vision, (2006) Circumcision no solution to AIDS – Museveni, 21 December 2006. Kampala: The New Vision publishing corporation,

Top ten tips on putting a communication strategy. (2007) [Online] ESRC. Available from the World Wide Web: <http://www.esrcsocietytoday.ac.uk/ESRCInfoCentre/Support/Communications_Toolkit/communications_strategy/top_ten_tips/> [Accessed 24 July 2007].

Towards a Universal access by 2010: How WHO is working with countries to scale up HIV prevention, treatment, care and support. (2006).[Online]. WHO. Available from the World Wide Web: <http://www.who.int/hiv/toronto2006/towardsuniversalaccess.pdf> [Accessed, 23 May 2007].

Tyndall, W.M.,Ronald,A.R.,Agoki,E.,malisa, W.,Bwayo,J.J., Ndunya-Achola,J.O.,Moses,S and Plummer, A.F. (1996) Increased risk of infection with Human Immunodeficiency virus type 1 among uncircumcised men presenting with genital ulcer disease in Kenya. *Clinical infectious diseases*. 23(3) 449-53.

Uganda HIV and AIDS Estimates. (2007) [Online] UNAIDS. Available from the World Wide Web: <http://www.unaids.org/en/Regions_Countries/Countries/Uganda.asp/> [Accessed 28th May 2007].

Ugandan men getting circumcised. (2007) [Online]. BBC. Available from the World Wide Web <http://news.bbc.co.uk/2/hi/africa/6227533.stm> [Accessed 7 February 2007].

UNAIDS/WHO fact sheet on male circumcision. (2007a) [Online]. UNAIDS. Available from the World Wide Web: <http://data.unaids.org/pub/FactSheet/2007/20061229_mc_fs_en.pdf> [Accessed 24. February 2007].

USAID/AIDSMARK (2000) Male Circumcision: Current Epidemiological and Field Evidence; Program and Policy Implications for HIV Prevention and Reproductive Health. Conference Report. Washington, DC: USAID, May 2003.

Wakabi,W. (2006) Condoms still contentious in Uganda's struggle over AIDS. *The Lancet* [Online] 367(9520), 1387- 1388. Available from World Wide Web: <http://0-www.sciencedirect.com.wam.leeds.ac.uk/> [5 April 2007].

Walt,G. (1994) Health Policy: An Introduction to process and power. Johannesburg: Witwatersrand University press.

Weiss, A.,Quigley,A.M.,Hayes,J.R (2000) Male circumcision and risk of HIV infection in sub- Saharan Africa: a systematic review and meta-analysis. *AIDS* [Online] 14(15), 2361-2370. Available from World Wide Web: <http://0-gateway.uk.ovid.com.wam.leeds.ac.uk/> [07 July 2007].

What is the situation of orphans and vulnerable children in Uganda? (2007) [Online]. The Republic of Uganda. Available from the World Wide Web: <http://www.mglsd.go.ug/ovc/Indicators.htm> [21 May 2007].

Wise,J. (2006) Demand for male circumcision rises in a bid to prevent HIV. *Bulletin of World Health organization* [Online]. 84(7), 509-511. Available from the World Wide Web : <http://www.who.int/bulletin/volumes/84/7/news.pdf> [23 March 2007].

Wiswell, E.T.,Smith,F.R & Bass,J.W. (1985) Decreased Incidence of Urinary Tract Infections in Circumcised Male Infants. *Pediatrics*[Online] 75(5), 901-903. Available from World Wide Web: <http://pediatrics.aappublications.org/cgi/reprint/75/5/901> [6 July 2007].

Wolff,B.,Nyanzi,B.,Katongole,G.,Ssesanga,D.,Ruberantwari,A.,Whitworth,J. (2005) Evaluation of a home-based voluntary counselling and testing intervention in rural Uganda *Health Policy Plan* [Online] 20(2), 109–116.Available from World Wide Web: <http://heapol.oxfordjournals.org/cgi/reprint/20/2/109/> [29 July 2007].

APPENDIX I – Search Methods for Other Sections

Database	Search Words	Total counts
Pubmed	**1.**Abstinence HIV/AIDS	307
	2.Be faithful	243
	3.Condoms HIV/AIDS	2680
	4.Voluntary counselling and testing	712
	5.Sexually transmitted infections	22012
	6.Sexually transmitted diseases	202360
	7.Uganda	5355
	8.Male protection	39228
	9.HIV/AIDS	107724
	10. Information, education, communication	10151
Combinations	1 and 7	269
	3 and 8	161
	10, 9 and 7	19
Global Health	HIV infections, Uganda with/or men, sexual behaviour Condom	399
	"Sexually transmitted infections" or "Sexually transmitted infections" "Uganda" Costs HIV access"	68

APPENDIX II
THE MONITOR NEWSPAPER COMMENT

Careful on circumcision

THE way the message on male circumcision is being expressed will become very significant in exploiting the benefits of male circumcision to reduce HIV infection in men. For example, your article, "Government calls for mass male circumcision", Daily Monitor, June 8 quoting Dr Zaramba that "We have data in Uganda, Kenya, South Africa that is very clear that circumcision substantially reduces the risk of a man contracting HIV through sexual intercourse and this is what we are advocating for" seems to front circumcision in its entirety in the prevention of HIV infection.

The media should champion better information, education and communication in promoting male circumcision and condom use. If this is done early enough, the strategy will realise a better protective effect. We are aware that male circumcision is not 100% effective against HIV infection.

But I am worried that although areas like Bugisu where male circumcision is a predominant cultural practice; there have been indications of 4.3% HIV prevalence compared to 3.6 % in Buganda among circumcised men in those areas (UHSBS, 2006). What could explain that higher prevalence in Bugisu?

If we do not begin by telling people right now that circumcision blends effectively with condom use, then we are in for the greatest HIV disaster. There is no way we are going to stop men from going on a rampage if they perceive that they are safe without their fore skin.

I have also noted that, unlike women, it is very hard to convince men to respond to existing voluntary counselling and testing facilities. This would be a good catch point for telling them the benefits of repackaged information for HIV prevention inclusive of male circumcision. If they are not told that after circumcision, they will have a 40% chance of contracting HIV, the efforts for circumcision would be wasted.

I like the approach of neonatal male circumcision in public hospitals proposed in the South Africa conference last week. The children would grow up having that 60% protective effect, but then also be educated with the ABC as they grow up. In that line of thinking, the Abstain, be faithful, condomise and circumcise (ABCC) strategy proposed by Uganda's Ministry of Health would be a very appropriate intervention.

James Kityo Ssemmanda,

University of Leeds, UK.

Source: Daily Monitor (Uganda). Published as, 'Today's pick', Letters to the Editor, June 11, 2007. Kampala: The Monitor Publications Ltd

Appendix III
UGANDA, HIV PREVALENCE BY REGION

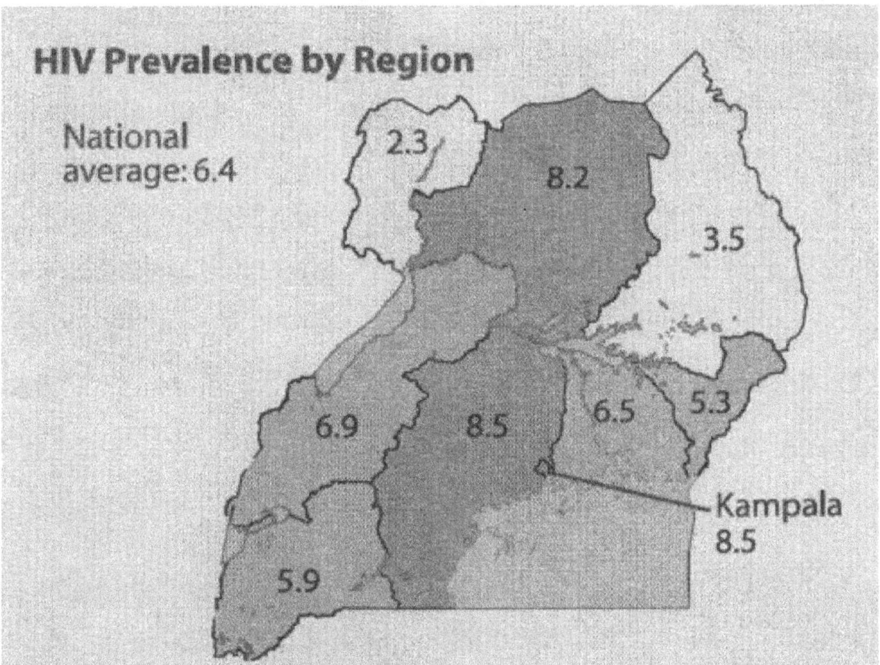

HIV prevalence is highest in Kampala (8.5 percent) and Central (8.5 percent). West Nile (2.3 percent) and Northeast (3.5 percent) have the lowest HIV prevalence.

Source: UHSBS (2006), Summary of data.

APPENDIX IV
OWNERSHPI OF HEALTH FACILITIES

DISTRICT	COUNTY	S/COUNTY	PARISH	No. HU's	P/HU's (+)	P/HU's (-)	% COVER	REQ. HU's
ADJUMANI	1	6	17	34	13	4	76.47	1
APAC	4	22	112	37	33	79	29.46	57
ARUA	8	37	225	62	65	167	28.89	115
BUGIRI	3	15	53	32	29	24	54.72	13
BUNDIBUGYO	2	10	38	20	20	18	52.63	10
BUSHENYI	7	30	156	66	61	95	39.10	64
BUSIA	1	10	34	20	16	18	47.06	11
GULU	5	23	122	46	44	78	36.07	54
HOIMA	2	13	51	37	33	18	64.71	8
IGANGA	4	25	137	102	87	50	63.50	23
JINJA	4	9	48	66	48	0	100.00	0
KABALE	4	19	119	68	63	56	52.94	32
KABAROLE	3	14	63	29	29	34	46.03	21
KABERAMAIDO	2	8	30	13	11	19	36.67	13
KALANGALA	2	7	17	9	9	8	52.94	5
KAMPALA	5	7	97	890	97	0	100.00	0
KAMULI	4	23	132	55	48	84	36.36	58
KAMWENGE	2	8	48	14	13	35	27.08	25
KANUNGU	1	8	50	17	17	33	34.00	23
KAPCHORWA	3	10	54	18	18	36	33.33	25
KASESE	2	21	105	65	48	57	45.71	36
KATAKWI	3	14	78	24	24	54	30.77	38
KAYUNGA	2	9	58	16	13	45	22.41	33
KIBAALE	3	18	65	34	28	37	43.08	24
KIBOGA	1	14	65	34	28	37	43.08	24
KISORO	1	14	36	13	13	23	36.11	16
KITGUM	2	13	64	21	21	43	32.81	30
KOTIDO	3	20	95	46	54	41	56.84	22
KUMI	3	16	107	30	24	81	22.43	62
KYENJOJO	3	14	79	31	30	49	37.97	33
LIRA	6	28	153	49	45	108	29.41	77

LUWERO	4	21	135	61	57	78	42.22	51
MASAKA	4	23	101	60	51	50	50.50	30
MASINDI	4	14	45	47	33	12	73.33	3
MAYUGE	1	6	37	27	26	11	70.27	4
MBALE	4	31	107	46	45	62	42.06	41
MBARARA	8	46	223	76	73	150	32.74	105
MOROTO	6	20	90	22	24	66	26.67	48
MOYO	2	8	23	28	17	6	73.91	1
MPIGI	3	17	118	42	40	78	33.90	54
MUBENDE	4	20	129	68	61	68	47.29	42
MUKONO	4	28	136	49	34	102	25.00	75
NAKAPIRIPIRIT	3	10	43	15	16	29	37.21	18
NAKASONGOLA	1	0	45	23	24	21	53.33	12
NEBBI	3	19	84	45	40	44	47.62	27
NTUNGAMO	3	14	84	25	25	59	29.76	42
PADER	2	13	53	20	19	34	35.85	23
PALLISA	4	22	80	42	38	42	47.50	26
RAKAI	4	26	115	47	45	70	39.13	47
RUKUNGIRI	2	11	70	25	23	47	32.86	33
SEMBABULE	2	7	33	12	9	24	27.27	17
SIRONKO	2	17	60	31	25	35	41.67	23
SOROTI	4	17	66	28	23	43	34.85	30
TORORO	5	21	71	40	35	36	49.30	22
WAKISO	2	15	130	50	37	93	28.46	67
YUMBE	1	8	32	12	14	18	43.75	12

APPENDIX V
CONDOMS – CONFIDENCE BUILDING MEASURE

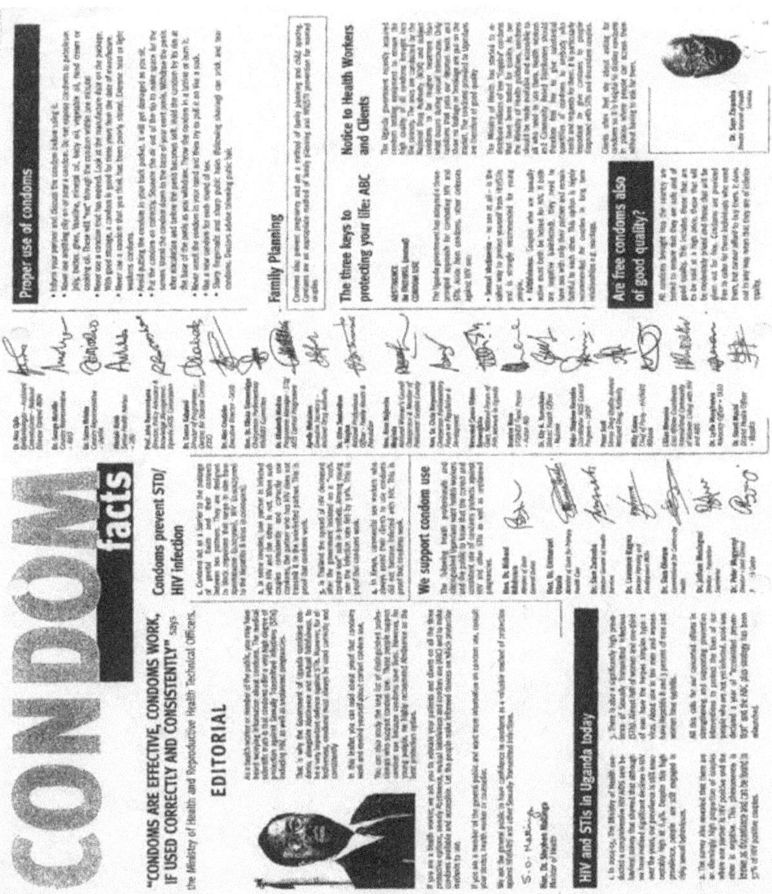

CONDOM facts

"CONDOMS ARE EFFECTIVE, CONDOMS WORK, IF USED CORRECTLY AND CONSISTENTLY" says the Ministry of Health and Reproductive Health Technical Officers.

EDITORIAL

Condoms prevent STD/ HIV infection

We support condom use

HIV and STIs in Uganda today

Proper use of condoms

Family Planning

The three keys to protecting your life: ABC

Notice to Health Workers and Clients

Are free condoms also of good quality?

Source: Ministry of Health, Uganda

www.ingramcontent.com/pod-product-compliance
Lightning Source LLC
LaVergne TN
LVHW010622300926
849162LV00001B/29